THE NATURE OF OUR HUMANITY

# THE NATURE OF OUR HUMANITY

## Ethical Issues in Genetics and Biotechnology

PAUL JERSILD

Fortress Press
Minneapolis

THE NATURE OF OUR HUMANITY
Ethical Issues in Genetics and Biotechnology

Copyright © 2009 Fortress Press, an imprint of Augsburg Fortress. All rights reserved. Except for brief quotations in critical articles or reviews, no part of this book may be reproduced in any manner without prior written permission from the publisher. Visit http://www.augsburgfortress.org/copyrights/ or write to Permissions, Augsburg Fortress, Box 1209, Minneapolis, MN 55440.

Scripture quotations from the New Revised Standard Version of the Bible are copyright © 1989 by the Division of Christian Education of the National Council of Churches of Christ in the United States of America and are used by permission.

Cover design: Joe Vaughan
Book design: PerfecType, Nashville, TN

*Library of Congress Cataloging-in-Publication data*

Jersild, Paul T., 1931–
  The nature of our humanity : ethical issues in genetics and biotechnology / by Paul Jersild.
     p. cm.
  Includes index.
  ISBN 978-0-8006-6442-8 (alk. paper)
  1. Theological anthropology—Christianity. 2. Bioethics—Religious aspects—Christianity. I. Title.
  BT702.J47 2009
  241'.64957—dc22
                                                2009006097

The paper used in this publication meets the minimum requirements for American National Standard for Information Sciences—Permanence of Paper for Printed Library Materials, ANSI Z329.48-1984.

Manufactured in the U.S.A.

This book is dedicated to my six grandchildren—
Annika, Kirsten, Emma, Olivia, Erika, and Maya—
who are sure to experience dimensions of biotechnological advance
that their grandfather can hardly imagine.

# CONTENTS

| | |
|---|---|
| Preface | ix |
| Introduction | xi |

**PART ONE: Christian Faith and Our Biological Past**

1. The Emergent Human Being — 3
   - Relating Faith to Evolutionary Biology — 4
   - Relating Evolutionary Biology to Faith — 13
   - To Be Human Is to Be in Relationship — 15
   - Biological Evolution and Human Nature — 20
   - Reconceptualizing the Soul — 23
   - Concluding Thoughts — 28

2. Human Nature and Biological Reductionism — 31
   - Scientific Materialism — 32
   - The Response of Intelligent Design — 37
   - A Critique of Scientific Materialism — 41
   - Searching for the Biological Basis of Religion — 46
   - Concluding Thoughts — 51

3. Human Nature and the Gene — 55
   - From Mendel to Watson and Crick — 56
   - Structure and Function of DNA — 57
   - Continuing Questions about the Gene — 59

| | |
|---|---:|
| The Human Genome Project | 62 |
| Interaction of Organism and Environment | 65 |
| A God Gene? | 69 |
| Genes, Culture, and Faith in God | 71 |
| Concluding Thoughts | 75 |

## PART TWO: Christian Faith and Our Biotech Future

### 4. Human Nature and the Impact of Biotechnology — 81
| | |
|---|---:|
| Theses Concerning Human Nature | 82 |
| Defining Biotechnology | 85 |
| Developments in Biotechnology | 88 |
| Creating a Superior Human Being | 93 |
| The Human Machine? | 97 |
| Scenarios of the Future | 100 |
| Concluding Thoughts | 103 |

### 5. Human Nature and Genetic Engineering — 107
| | |
|---|---:|
| What Is Genetic Engineering? | 108 |
| From Therapy to Enhancement | 111 |
| The Enhancement Argument | 115 |
| The Anti-enhancement Argument | 119 |
| Human Nature and the Human Future | 129 |
| Concluding Thoughts | 132 |

### 6. Human Nature and the Quest for Immortality — 137
| | |
|---|---:|
| Living with the Prospect of Death | 138 |
| The Controversial Embryonic Stem Cell | 141 |
| Stem Cells, Telomeres, and the Life Span | 147 |
| Other Aging Factors | 150 |
| Biblical Insights on Human Mortality | 152 |
| A Critique of the Immortality Quest | 160 |
| Concluding Thoughts | 163 |

| | |
|---|---:|
| Notes | 167 |
| Index | 185 |

# PREFACE

Writing this book has occasioned a serendipitous occurrence, bringing me together with a remarkable physician, now in his nineties, who has been a leader in reproductive technology. Howard Jones is a nephew of the well-known missionary and writer E. Stanley Jones, who together with his late wife shepherded to birth the first baby in the United States conceived through in vitro fertilization. Apart from the joy and fulfillment he and his associates have brought to many hundreds of infertile couples, Dr. Jones has contributed substantially to a biomedical field that is directly related to the subject matter of this book. I mention him here because of his gracious willingness to read most of its chapters, providing valuable suggestions along the way.

Another acquaintance made as a result of writing this book is Barbara King, professor of anthropology at William and Mary College. I have profited from conversation with her as well as from her published work. One biologist in particular has been quite helpful to me: Professor Maynard Schaus of Virginia Wesleyan College. I also want to acknowledge the helpful critique of the first chapter by Hans Tiefel, professor emeritus at William and Mary. Last but not least, I am thankful for the supportive interest of my sister, Joann Spiegel, who as a former editor was able to offer helpful suggestions on grammar and style as well as content, based on her own considerable reading on the cutting edges of genetics and biotechnology.

Finally, a sincere word of appreciation to Michael West, Susan Johnson, and Sheila Anderson of Fortress Press for their assistance and competence in bringing this book to completion.

# INTRODUCTION

This book addresses subject matter that turns the reader in two opposite directions, and for that reason, it is divided into two parts. Part one turns us to the past, raising the question "Who are we?" in light of our origins as human beings. This involves a consideration of biological evolution and how it can be incorporated into the Christian's understanding of human nature. It also brings a Christian response to the philosophical materialism that often poses as a necessary accompaniment of biological and genetic assessments of the human being. Part two turns us to the future and once again raises the question "Who are we?" but now in light of the future impact of biotechnology. Particular attention will be given to efforts at genetic enhancement, including strategies for overcoming human mortality. In light of projections being made by microbiologists and bioengineers, what changes lie in store for the human community, what will they mean for the future identity of human beings, and how are we to respond to these possible developments as Christians? These questions will become increasingly urgent in coming years with the growing impact of technological advance; the frontiers of biotechnology are being continually pushed back in the quest for greater control over our minds and our bodies.

Throughout the centuries, theologians have reflected at length on the distinctive features of a Christian understanding of human nature, always in response to the cultural currents that have influenced their times. The era in which we now live is particularly challenging in light of scientific and technological developments that appear to threaten traditional Christian understandings of who we are. Any reflection today on this subject matter—what we call "theological anthropology"—must therefore address the biosciences and biotechnology if it is to be relevant and helpful to the Christian community. If the church's theologians are adequately carrying out their task, they will have one foot firmly planted in their tradition and the other just as firmly planted in the culture of their own time, which for us is deeply influenced by the mind-set of science and technology. It is a conversational enterprise that requires openness on the part of theologians to the cutting edges of their culture as well as discernment of where and how those edges should be challenged or affirmed. A critical part of this discussion is identifying the genuine problems and challenges that mark the divide between science and religion, and avoiding the creation of false differences and unnecessary tensions.

It is instructive to reflect on this ongoing cultural conversation between science and religion and the different shape it has taken in succeeding centuries. In the sixteenth and seventeenth centuries, the emerging science of astronomy challenged the reigning Ptolemaic view of the cosmos, which served the church's teaching by placing the earth at the center of God's universe. Humanity, after all, was at the center of God's attention, and the cosmos reflected that fact. The theories of Copernicus and Galileo brought a profound shock to this thinking; quite understandably, there was considerable resistance, and throughout the seventeenth century, it was common for universities (Harvard, for example) to teach both the Ptolemaic and Copernican views side by side. What was taking place was not just a scientific debate, but a religious and cultural struggle. It took time for people of faith to reassess their understanding of the cosmos, but that reassessment happened long ago, and the church has adjusted to it. Astronomy is not the final authority when it comes to defining who we are as human beings.

From the late nineteenth century to our own times, the principal scientific threat to Christian self-understanding undoubtedly has been the theory of biological evolution identified with Charles Darwin (1809–1882). This theory has been a significant challenge to the church, because its impact on our understanding of who we are has been more personal and immediate. Given the intense negative reaction to Darwinism in many Christian circles to this day, most people are surprised to learn that already in the nineteenth century, there were notable theologians who responded positively to Darwin's concept of biological evolution. Some incorporated it into their theology as a framework for understanding God's relation to the world, or "God's way of doing things." Such was the view of the Reverend Charles Kingsley, chaplain to Queen Victoria and a respected intellectual of his time, who acknowledged in a letter to Darwin that his book, *The Origin of Species* (1859), had compelled him to reassess his understanding of God's relation to the world. One of the more conservative theologians of the time, Benjamin B. Warfield of Princeton Theological Seminary, accepted evolution as "a theory of the method of divine providence," arguing the necessity of a divine author behind the process of evolution.[1] Darwin himself refers to the grandeur of biological evolution in the conclusion of *The Origin of Species*: "with its several powers having been originally breathed by the Creator into a few forms or into one." In his later years, he acknowledged that agnosticism was closest to his "state of mind"; he didn't regard biological evolution as offering a definitive proof one way or the other as far as God was concerned.[2]

The latter half of the twentieth century saw an increasingly fruitful exchange between scientists and theologians, helping to forge a spirit of dialogue between their disciplines (unfortunately, a dialogue that is far removed from most of the public discussion). I have not been a part of that dialogue and do not have the credentials to contribute to it, but it provides a helpful background to a work of this kind. My focus is limited to a consideration of human nature, touching just incidentally on broader issues in the science-and-religion dialogue. A substantial part of my discussion (in chapters 2 and 3) will focus on philosophical and ideological arguments that too easily infiltrate what is identified as a "scientific worldview," causing much of the tension between scientific and religious assessments of human nature. This is not to deny that advocates on the religious side have also muddied the water with claims that strike many Christians today as obscurantist, showing disdain for scientific findings that have long found consensus in the scientific community.

Even though public polling in the United States on the subject of biological evolution has always revealed considerable resistance to it, there have been signs lately of a gradual easing of this conflict; I believe a significant percentage of the laity and clergy in the older denominations are ready to put this divisive struggle behind them. A recent indication of this fact has been the appearance of the Clergy Letter Project, a national campaign organized to counteract the influence of creationists and fundamentalist churches and to affirm the compatibility of religion and science. A special feature of its program is the Evolution Weekend, which by 2008 had grown to more than eight hundred congregations from every state of the union and nine foreign countries, all committed to devoting an annual worship observance or a class to the subject of evolution and a proper religious response to it. More than eleven thousand clergy members have signed a statement in support of evolutionary teaching. At its 2008 General Convention, the United Methodist Church added the acceptance of evolution to its *Book of Discipline*, stating, "We find that science's description of cosmological, geological, and biological evolution is not in conflict with theology."

The importance of the biosciences for theology has not been easy for theologians to accept. The cultural setting for theological anthropology has been largely shaped by philosophical currents quite apart from the findings of the natural sciences. Even where theologians have been open to the implications of the biosciences and specifically to the theory of biological evolution, many at best (myself included) have felt less than comfortable in permitting these subjects to influence their theology in meaningful ways. Yet any treatment of who we are as human beings has to recognize that we are rooted in the natural world and that our nature and identity cannot be understood apart from that reality. We are mortal beings, bound by the limitations of our bodily selves, and we are intimately related to the rest of the natural world, both animate and inanimate. By raising the question "Who are we?" specifically within the context of biological evolution and biological attempts to modify and "re-create" the human condition, we gain answers that are all the more fruitful and significant for us. Christian theology must dialogue with the biosciences simply because it is the responsible thing to do, but beyond this, it provides the opportunity to bring new insights to the understanding of our humanity and to the philosophical and moral issues we are facing.³

As we survey the contemporary scene, it is likely that recent developments in genetics and molecular biology are going to fuel one of the most intense and critical confrontations yet seen between science and religion. These developments involve the subject matter of part two, which raises issues that our ancestors could hardly have imagined. The reason for this is simple enough: the primary object of these scientific explorations is not the world "out there," but the inner world of humans themselves. The Human Genome Project has transformed our knowledge of human beings at the genomic level, and the ongoing inventions of computers and other machinery that enable scientists to study the human subject at the molecular level are opening up new dimensions of understanding. How the worlds of science and religion respond to these developments should be of interest to everyone; there is the potential to further alienate and divide these two worlds or to generate new and promising understandings that can deepen the respect of each for the other.

The current tensions, however, go well beyond the relation of science to religion. The handmaid of science is technology, which transforms the results of scientific research into a magnificent array of practical applications that serve the human community in countless ways. The capacity not only to study but also to manipulate and modify the human being at the genetic level is raising momentous ethical issues that will dominate the public discussion for years to come. Indeed, some of the most intense ethical issues of our time have literally been created by biomedical technology, and they apply quite directly to the issues I will be addressing in part two. Underlying these ethical issues are fundamental questions of human identity that are supremely important to the person of faith. "What should we do?" is a question that carries with it the deeper question "Who are we, and what is the purpose of human existence?" This question underlies the subject matter of this book.

My purpose in writing is to help particularly those in the Christian community to gain a better grasp of current developments in genetics and biotechnology and to help them forge an appropriate theological and ethical response. To do this at all adequately, I thought it necessary to discuss at some length the biological and genetic material that I am addressing, assuming also that most readers are not all that familiar with it. My professional education as a theologian and ethicist equips me for the theological dimensions of this work, but my limited background in the natural sciences has required an extensive (and, I must say, a most rewarding) reading program on genetics and biology in order to do justice to that dimension. I'm well aware of scientist-theologian John Polkinghorne's comment that "theologians often do not achieve great sophistication or insight when they turn to science," nor for that matter do scientists when they turn to theology, but he is quick to acknowledge that "the moral is not that we should all return to the comfort and safety of our professional home grounds."[4] While interdisciplinary work is inherently risky, theologians still need to be doing it for the sake of the church's witness in the world. It is a task that requires humility and openness to what we can learn, as well as confidence that we bring a perspective that needs to be heard.

There are many "battlegrounds" where science and religion have come into conflict, but certainly the central one has been the status of the human being. My primary task has been to lift up a theological and anthropological perspective that is rooted in the Christian revelation and to relate it to the findings in genetics and biology. What does our creation "in the image of God" mean in relation to our biological heritage, and what does that heritage have to say to us in understanding the image of God? What can we learn from the new genetics about ourselves, and what conclusions and inferences are to be drawn from that knowledge? What constitutes responsible interpretation of the results of genetic investigations as they relate to larger issues of human meaning and destiny? Part one in particular addresses these questions in forging a Christian view of human nature; the reader will find a summary of my conclusions at the beginning of chapter 4 before I turn to the subject of biotechnology.

As a forecast of what is to come and to give the reader a preliminary indication of my own stance, I mention here some of the themes that will play an important role in the pages that follow. My basic thesis concerning the current conflict between science and religion, governed on the scientific side by genetics and molecular biology, is that it is a philosophical debate that involves flawed assumptions and inferences on both sides. In every chapter, I will be challenging what I call a "genocentric" or reductionist view of human nature that replaces the macro world of human relationships with the micro world of molecular activity as a source of explanation for who we are as human beings. Central to my understanding of human nature is the fact that we are relational beings, with our relation to God and to each other making our humanity possible. This understanding establishes community as the goal of human life, a goal that captures the meaning and promise of life together. It also takes our bodily character seriously, recognizing the biological rootedness of our spiritual life and insisting on the holistic character of our nature, in contrast to the dualism of body and soul that has dominated the Christian tradition. I bring these understandings to the consideration of the ethical and theological issues raised by biotechnology, particularly the challenges of genetic enhancements and attempts to overcome human mortality.

Each of these themes warrants a book in itself, but I hope the overall picture I present will be helpful for inquiring readers in developing their own theological and ethical stance, as well as whet their appetite for further reading on the issues that are raised. I also hope this work contributes to the education of the church, equipping it to address issues that are critically important both for its own life and for that of the larger society.

# PART ONE

# CHRISTIAN FAITH AND OUR BIOLOGICAL PAST

CHAPTER 1

# The Emergent Human Being

The questions "Who are we?" and "Why are we here?" have been a central part of Christian theology, requiring clear and perceptive answers on the basis of the biblical revelation. A critical factor in answering these questions is the cultural setting, which gives form and shape to the questions asked and the answers given. Living in a culture that has been profoundly shaped by the scientific and technological revolutions of the modern age, we cannot address these questions without recognizing the impact of the natural sciences, particularly the biological sciences. The theory of biological evolution stands prominently in the cultural environment in which the Christian theologian works, and consequently must be addressed in any reflections having to do with human nature and identity.[1] This fact is a reminder of the evolving character of theology itself, simply because it does not occur in a vacuum but in conversation with its culture. The gospel of Jesus Christ remains the same, but it will not be heard as good news if it is not interpreted in light of the times.

To bring together the biological and theological dimensions of human nature is to use two quite different paradigms in addressing the same human subject. My thesis is that these two paradigms are complementary to each other (which is to say they "complete" each other), with each claiming a particular competence in addressing human nature, each bringing its own particular assumptions and methodology to the subject, and each bringing an indispensable perspective to a complete understanding of the human being. Science brings an empirical mindset, seeking answers within the bounds allowed by empirical investigation—what are often characterized as the "what" questions. Religion, by contrast, focuses on larger questions concerning meaning and destiny—the "why" questions that raise transcendent issues and invite a faith commitment. My purpose is to propose a Christian understanding of human nature that relates positively to biological evolution and captures the essential features of a Christian anthropology. Rather than addressing this subject in a comprehensive manner, I want to propose a way of reconceptualizing our understanding of human nature and the image of God in light of biological evolution.

## Relating Faith to Evolutionary Biology

In addressing human nature, the Christian theologian proceeds from the biblical revelation, a narrative concerning the Hebrew people that culminates for the Christian in the story of Jesus of Nazareth. This piece of history from ancient times provides the substance for the Christian's understanding of who we are as human beings, reflecting the belief that the ultimate word concerning human nature and destiny is to be found in history rather than in nature. Nature provides the indispensable setting for the story, and it necessarily enters into that story in a variety of ways, but historical action is what brings meaning to what humanity is all about. Because this story is an ancient one, its references to the world of nature reflect an ancient cosmology, far removed from our knowledge of the world and from the ways in which we relate to the world in an age of technology.

With this background, it is difficult indeed for Christians to face the reality that our relation to nature has become decisive for our faith in God and for our self-understanding as human beings. We understand today as never before that all of our thinking and doing as biological selves are profoundly influenced and conditioned by nature.

Darwin's theory of biological evolution, including his thesis that natural selection ("the survival of the fittest") is the most likely means by which the world's species emerge and disappear, has become an essential feature of the scientific understanding of the biological world. As the Christian geneticist Theodor Dobzhansky observed, "Nothing in biology makes sense except in the light of evolution."[2] Thus, we are challenged as never before to integrate our understanding of God's relation to the world and of our own human nature with the knowledge of the biosciences. The biblical story is not replaced in this venture, nor is a scientific discipline placed on a pedestal so that it supersedes our affirmations of faith. Rather, we are willing to recognize that the Bible and Christian tradition can and should be interpreted in a way that allows us to acknowledge and critically affirm what has been universally established as truth in the scientific community. It is of course true that the sciences as heuristic disciplines are always in a state of development and change, but nevertheless, there is a body of evidence that provides the foundations for further inquiry and that warrants the respect of the theologian.

In the paragraphs that follow, I will briefly sketch some of the major topics (*loci*) of Christian theology, affirming a Christian theistic position in conversation with biological evolution. My purpose is to suggest a contemporary Christian basis for understanding the human being in light of the biosciences before expanding later in the chapter on some of the implications of these statements.

## *God the Creator*

Christians confess their faith in God as "Creator of heaven and earth," a confession based on the biblical story that begins with the creation account (actually two accounts) in Genesis 1–2. It is a story of remarkable literary quality and theological depth, but unfortunately a story that has itself posed a large part of the problem in the conflict between science and religion. Until quite recent times, most Christians assumed that the Genesis story was one coherent and descriptive account of what happened when the world came into being. This has meant that the beginning chapters of Genesis have been pitted against the developing knowledge of science concerning human origins, as though the two were comparable as accounts of the beginning of things.

We now live in a time when Christians in significant numbers are able to recognize that the Bible contains a variety of literary genres, which means that the test of the Bible's veracity is not whether all that it relates is true in a literal sense. The discerning reader finds a wealth of different materials in the Bible: stories such as parables, allegories, and myths that convey a moral or theological point, as well as a fair amount of historical reporting, moral exhortation, hymns, poetry, proverbs, and legendary material. Throughout history, Christians have typically regarded the biblical story of creation as a kind of newspaper account of what happened; for most people living prior to the Age of Enlightenment, there was neither the knowledge nor the motivation to question the authoritative tradition of religion and culture on a matter of this kind. With the emergence of the scientific age and greater sophistication in assessing the subject of the world's origin, Christians can recognize the creation account for what it is: a story inspired by faith that introduces the larger biblical story of salvation and sets the stage for God's relationship to the creation and particularly to humanity. It is a *religious* story, organized around the sacred week and using a literary pattern for each day that glorifies the creative acts of God. Whether one lives in ancient or modern times, the only way one can address the subject of creation is to tell a story, because the subject transcends history.

One of the ironies in the literalist view of the creation story that has held such a tenacious grip on the popular mind is that the basis for a proper understanding is found already in ancient times among leading theologians of the church. Writing in 231 C.E., the Greek theologian Origen noted, concerning certain expressions in the early chapters of Genesis, "I do not think anyone will doubt that these are figurative expressions which indicate mysteries through a semblance of history." In his commentary on Genesis (391 C.E.), Augustine wrote concerning chapter 1: "No Christian would dare say that the narrative must not be taken in a figurative sense."[3] Today we recognize that the creation story moves us beyond the time-bound to the realm of myth, expressing in story form a profound truth about the meaning of things. It conveys the truth that God is the author of all things, quite apart from offering a scientific description of *how* the world or the human species came into being. There is a world of difference between a creation story and a scientific account of the origin of things.

Unfortunately, the challenge for much Christian theology still today is to recognize this difference and to acknowledge that theology has something to learn from the natural sciences. Where this has occurred, we see an understanding of creation that shifts from disparate acts of God back at the beginning of things (the elements of a mythic story) to God as eternal Creator, creating continuously. This is not a denial of *creatio ex nihilo* (creation out of nothing), for God supersedes the creation, but it is an affirmation of *creatio continua* (continuing creation) in understanding the unfolding nature of creation. Biological evolution dramatizes the fact that the world itself is an epic story that involves the capacity to bring forth what is new. As William Temple, archbishop of Canterbury, noted a century ago, "God did not make things . . . no, but He made them make themselves."[4] When we bring creation and evolution together, we do not look for some kind of miraculous beginning that would confirm a creative act of God. Instead, this approach commits us to a thoroughly naturalistic understanding of what we can learn about the origin of things. We are not looking for divine acts along the way (which have often been proposed to fill in the "gaps" of our scientific knowledge) but can marvel at the capacity of nature to bring forth an evolving pattern of life. We affirm as an act of faith that God brings into being and continues to sustain this whole process that generates the emergence of self-organizing systems and of organic life, including the comparatively recent development of human life. The beginnings of life remain shrouded in mystery, but a mystery that Christians can freely acknowledge together with the conviction that the evolutionary process is "God's way of doing things."

In recent times, the term *panentheism* (all is in God and God is in all, without exhausting God's presence to the creation) has been used to describe a Christian Trinitarian understanding that would stress God's immanence in the world more forcefully than the church's traditional theism. Informed by scientific and ecological concerns, panentheists are critical of the tendency to speak in monotheistic terms about the Father who creates the world, because this imagery tends to convey God's transcendence to the exclusion of God's immanence. While pantheism (identifying God with the world) is obviously to be rejected, a Trinitarian view leads us to emphasize the Spirit of God as God's presence in creation. When the apostle Paul, speaking to the Athenians, quoted approvingly the words of a Greek poet, "In him we live and move and have our being" (Acts 17:28), he was affirming the truth that God's Spirit is immediately present and active at every level of creation in which we move. In light of the biblical revelation, the divine mystery is naturally expressed in terms of personal relationship and personal agency within human history. But at the same time, the immanence of God relates to the whole of life, including God's creative activity in the world of nature and the ongoing process of bringing forth what is new. As expressed by theologian Jürgen Moltmann:

> Everything that is, exists and lives in the unceasing inflow of the energies and potentialities of the cosmic Spirit. This means that we have to understand every created reality in terms of energy, grasping it as the realized potentiality of the divine Spirit. Through the energies and potentialities of the Spirit, the Creator is himself present in his creation.[5]

Christians who would bring their faith into conversation with science are bound to hear the accusation "Your God is too small!" To relate God to the world of nature and to the staggering scope of the universe itself compels us to move beyond the anthropomorphisms we commonly hear among Christians. The "man upstairs" notion of God, with which we are all too familiar, only trivializes a concept that should convey overwhelming mystery. Because of the biblical revelation and particularly the mission and message of Jesus, we know God as personal presence, but as the divine Spirit, God transcends human personhood and eludes every attempt to define and grasp the divine. That is reason for humility and a reminder of our limitations as created beings, as well as a reminder that the world of science can help to keep us responsible in the language we use when speaking of God.

## *The Emergent Human Being*

The Christian narrative focuses on human beings as God's children with a divinely bestowed destiny. This includes a further truth about who we are, expressed in two passages from the book of Genesis: "Then the LORD God formed man from the dust of the ground" (2:7), and "You are dust, and to dust you shall return" (3:19). Humans are clearly related to the whole of God's world, sharing in the larger story of nature itself. The Hebrew word in the book of Genesis from which we derive the name of Adam is *adamah*, meaning literally "from the earth." The elements of the "primordial soup" from which all of God's creatures emerge continue to constitute the human being as well as the whole organic and inorganic world. Whether one is speaking of human beings, flies, plants, bacteria, or fungi, all share in the genetic structure of life; DNA (deoxyribonucleic acid), the chemical basis of heredity, is a common thread in relating all of life. Christian theology is thus obligated to place human beings firmly in the midst of God's natural world; while our capacity to manipulate and shape the environment gives us a unique status in bearing responsibility for the creation, we remain members of the animal kingdom and subject to all the limitations of that reality.

We might say there is a paradoxical character to human nature, in which we are children of God with an eternal destiny but also creatures who share the mortality that marks all of God's creatures. We live in a time when our connectedness to the rest of the animal world is becoming increasingly clear, shedding light on the biological nature of our existence. In the conversation between religion and science, it is imperative that we stress this twofold character of human identity in which we recognize and affirm the *continuity* of the human being with the animal kingdom at the same time that we recognize and affirm the *discontinuity*. This does not pose a contradiction that cannot be reconciled. It is, rather, a dialectical assertion that has to be made whenever we speak of the identity of human beings. We are by nature both creatures of God and creatures of the earth.

The emergence of life on earth can be seen as a marvel of awesome proportions, given the fact that it has required such a delicate balance in the wide variety of physical forces that constitute the universe. Had such elements as the mass of the universe, various particle masses, gravitational force, electromagnetic force, and the velocity of light, to name but a few, been only slightly different, the galaxies and planets would have been totally different, with no possibility of life developing on earth.[6] Some have called these coincidences that have made carbon-based life (and so human life) possible the "anthropic principle"; the universe is so finely tuned that it has generated, through its own inherent properties, living organisms and finally *Homo sapiens*. While this reality does not constitute a proof for the existence of God (as some would argue), it does contribute to the Christian's conviction that we live in the kind of world that can be intelligibly united with belief in God. Such belief does not require that we be able to identify "special acts" of God in the emerging creation, but it recognizes the propensities of the evolutionary process toward increase in complexity, consciousness, and finally self-consciousness.[7]

The emergence of self-consciousness brings into being a creature who reflects the image of God, who can relate to God and fellow human beings and begin to fulfill a God-given destiny. Though Christians tend to see the human being as the climax of creation, it is important to recognize that, scientifically speaking, the movement from simple to complex organization in itself does not *demonstrate* purpose and design. The emergence of *Homo sapiens* takes place in a process marked by contingency rather than inevitability, but this in turn does not rule out a creator. Some would claim that the element of randomness in biological evolution justifies the notion that the emergence of human beings has been purely accidental, but this is an exaggerated claim. We do not insist on inevitability and purposive direction in *human* history as assurance that God is in the process, and neither should we expect to find them in *natural* history.[8] Freedom and contingency within a context of order and structure are inherent to both nature and history.

## *Sin and the Fall*

In light of our rootedness in the natural world, it has been tempting for Christian theologians to explain human sinfulness in terms of our "animal nature," or the fact that we are creatures of instinct. To place human beings within the context of biological evolution would appear to accentuate this kind of thinking, leading one to believe that the human problem is due to our animal background that we are now challenged to transcend and overcome. On the contrary, Christian theology recognizes human sin as a spiritual condition, best described in terms of human pride and self-centeredness that go well beyond the natural instinct of self-preservation. With the emergence of self-consciousness in the human being has come the awareness of moral failure, guilt, and mortality. These defining dimensions of humanity from early on brought an awareness of transcendence and efforts to secure one's life by acts of appeasement directed to the gods. Thus, moral evil that compromises and destroys human relationships is understood as sin that incurs divine judgment. In securing ourselves in the face of our vulnerabilities, we make a competitor and enemy of our neighbor and challenge the divine order that sustains life itself.

In recognizing sin as a state or condition, the Christian understanding sheds considerable light on the human situation. Our problem is not the result of individual transgressions but betrays a state of being that gives rise to transgression. An evolutionary understanding sees both our biological and cultural heritage playing into this predicament, not in any deterministic way but as setting the context and conditions in which humans in their freedom respond to the demands of life. Some have understood human evolution to be a steady course of moral progress from an animal past, but the evidence would indicate a far more ambiguous picture. In many respects, a more civilized society does emerge with the evolution of cultures, but there is ample evidence that evolving societies invent still more horrific ways to exalt themselves and destroy their neighbors. Evolution, whether biological or cultural, does not mean inexorable progress on the road toward perfection. However, it does constitute a genuine alternative to the church's traditional view of the fall, which asserts that humans were originally in a state of innocence and then experienced a fall into sin by virtue of the initial sin by Adam. Given the mythical character of this story, Christian theology today has generally moved beyond this traditional view; holding to an evolutionary view of an emergent humanity would also require the rejection of a historical understanding of the fall, including the fact that there is no biological-historical evidence for such a transition. Adam is recognized as a representative rather than a historical figure, standing not at the beginning of history but in the midst of each of our histories, signifying the human problem with which we struggle.

## *Redemption in Jesus the Christ*

Jesus, the Christ or chosen one of God, is central to the faith of the church, the one in whom God makes God's self known in a once-for-all, decisive manner. This revelation is centered in the life and activity of Jesus: as a result of his ministry, he was acclaimed as the long-awaited Messiah; in his message and accompanying "works of wonder," he proclaimed and embodied the coming of the kingdom of God; his compassionate life embraced all members of society, even "the least of these," the poor and the despised; his speaking truth to religious and political power led him to a criminal's death on a cross; and his death was followed by the mystery of the resurrection. The profound impact of this train of events led quite early to reflection on Jesus' relation to the God whom he called "Father," leading eventually to the church's confession that Jesus is both "true man" and "true God." This language from the Council of Chalcedon (451 C.E.) expresses the church's understanding concerning the meaning of Jesus' life: God was at work in what Jesus did and in what happened to him.

By placing the Christian understanding of Jesus within the context of evolution, we become aware of the close connection between the historical setting of his life and the material, biological world in which God is continually giving existence to what is new. The creative process is built into the very process of evolution, in which an evolving matter brings forth new levels of complexity. This process has resulted in mental and spiritual qualities that distinguish human beings, placing them in relation to God and consequently revealing in themselves the image of God. This image appears in Jesus as the consummation of God's purposes; he is the "new creation," the paradigm for the rest of humanity. But his meaning and significance are not limited to humanity. Scripture makes clear that the redemption he embodies is of cosmic scope, bringing an ultimate promise that embraces all of life, "things in heaven and things on earth" (Eph. 1:10). The seal of his being chosen by God for this life-giving purpose is the resurrection, which reveals both his redemptive role and the ultimate destiny of humanity. Thus, the church has been moved to see in Jesus God Incarnate, the one who embodies the will and purpose of God and through whom the Spirit brings forgiveness and new life.[9] Jesus puts "a human face" on God that enables the believer to approach God as a loving Father and to enter into a life of obedience in the spirit of Jesus himself. Clearly, this kind of affirmation is not simply an objective judgment based on historical information, but reflects the experience of believers who are addressed by the figure of Jesus as the embodiment of divine love and forgiveness.

These admittedly sketchy understandings of several cardinal Christian beliefs should indicate that a traditional Christian theological stance can be expressed within the context of evolutionary biology. Bringing these two disciplines together can both enrich our understanding of the faith and convey the relevance of that faith to the scientific world. The latter point should be made with a proper sense of humility; we do not use science to prove the validity of the faith, but to assert that believers recognize that their faith is intelligible and can bring insight to the larger questions posed by human existence in a mystifying world. Making this venture of dialogue is the first step for the Christian in entering the larger conversation about the burning issues of the day, many of which are posed by the impact of the biosciences and the biotechnology they have spawned. A critical issue in this conversation is human nature and identity, a subject on which Christians have a most important contribution to make.

## Relating Evolutionary Biology to Faith

The reflections in the previous section bring theology and evolutionary biology together from the viewpoint of a theologian who expresses his faith in conversation with biology. Evolutionary biologists who are believers will see the point and importance of this venture, but in light of their discipline, both believing and unbelieving biologists will bring their particular perspective to the subject of religious faith, asking questions and seeking answers that reflect the interests of their discipline. Since the 1990s, there has been a notable increase in the attention that evolutionary biologists have given to religious faith; in particular, they seek an answer to the question "In the struggle for survival that marks evolution, what role does religious belief play?" The object of interest here (at least at a primary level) isn't whether religious experience is authentic or whether the notion of God points to a metaphysical reality. Instead, it represents an effort within a particular science to determine how religious belief fits into the process of natural selection.[10] Has belief in God assisted humanity to effectively adapt to its environment, or has it been a by-product or result of other adaptations during the course of evolution? Does religious belief serve humanity in what the believer would regard as our God-given destiny, to be stewards of creation, or should it be regarded as a neurological accident in the evolution of the brain that either hinders or has little to do with the flourishing of humanity?

Given the universality of religion, one could understandably conclude that it must have evolutionary value. If religious beliefs worked against an effective adaptation to the environment, would not the evolutionist have to wonder about their staying power? However, many religious beliefs appear to be what anthropologist Scott Atran calls "counter-intuitive," misunderstanding and misrepresenting the world. Animistic beliefs, for example, posit spirits as active agents that "explain" events in the natural world; humans have had to outgrow such notions in order to understand and to deal effectively with their natural environment. One obvious problem in gaining a handle on this subject is its diffuse character. Religious belief covers every conceivable aspect of human life, from understanding nature to figuring out the meaning of human existence, from relating to one's neighbor to projecting a human destiny. It is a life orientation that may include any number of mistaken ideas about matters that lie beyond our comprehension but also inspires a sense of meaning and purpose for one's personal life and creates a community that assists in providing coherence and direction for self and family. It may all be rooted in self-deception, or it may all be rooted in a profound truth that stands beyond the capacity of science to determine: we are all children of God.

How religious faith takes shape in people's lives, what responsibilities it leads them to assume, what risks it emboldens them to take—all of these have a bearing on the course of cultural evolution. Religious faith is a generic term that has to be related to the particular faiths by which people live, and one can surmise that those faiths that have persevered over centuries and millennia have served their adherents well in the struggle for survival. Wherever convictions of faith bring a sense of wholeness and purpose to life, compelling one to face the world with honesty and confidence, to reach out to the neighbor instead of succumbing to fear and alienation, to celebrate the universal human community rather than exalting tribalism—there the possibilities of human flourishing are enhanced. The continuing challenge for the historic religions is to lift up and to embody the ethical imperatives that reflect the direction of their convictions and the promise of humanity, recognizing that in serving God, we are serving each other and the welfare of God's world.

## To Be Human Is to Be in Relationship

In presenting an understanding of humanity, I have turned to the Bible and the God of the Bible—the Triune God whom Christians confess as Creator, Redeemer, and life-giving Spirit. At the center of this biblical faith is the conviction that, as creatures, we stand in covenantal relation to God, a reality that no human being or human institution can remove. This conviction has implications that need to be spelled out further, particularly the point that our "divine connectedness" supersedes all other distinctions we are prone to make in our understanding of humanity. Our relation to God embraces our relations with other human beings, and this reality is the foundation for who we are. Relationships are indispensable to our nature and identity as human beings, for we become who we are by being in relationship. Theologian Jürgen Moltmann makes this point by distinguishing between individuality and personhood:

An individual, like an atom, is literally that ultimate element of indivisibility. An ultimate element of indivisibility, however, has no relationships, and also cannot communicate. . . . By contrast, a person is the individual human being in the resonance field of the relationships of I-you-we, I-myself, I-it. Within this network of relationships, the person becomes the subject of giving and taking, hearing and doing, experiencing and touching, perceiving and responding. . . . The "person" emerges through the call of God.[11]

Moltmann's understanding of the "call of God" is a call into interpersonal relationship with God and other persons, making possible our self-knowledge and self-identity, all of which are inseparable.[12] Essential to our personhood and to our standing in relationship is the fact that we are bodily selves; we cannot know ourselves and others in this world without our bodily nature. To know ourselves as children of God is to recognize a relationship that defines human existence, establishing a fundamental orientation to life itself and to our relations with other human beings. Consequently, central to our understanding of human nature is our God-given capacity to relate to God as a covenantal partner and to other humans as fellow creatures. These relationships also place us in a position of responsibility to the surrounding world, to fulfill the divine command to rule over and to care for the world in ways that fulfill our destiny as "created co-creators" with God.[13] This capacity and all it implies are what we mean by the expression *image of God*, a central biblical concept that has received a variety of interpretations in Christian theology.

Despite the variety, one can identify two dominant understandings of the image of God in the history of Christian thought. The most prominent view, seen in the Roman Catholic tradition today and going back to the church fathers, can be characterized as "substantialist," in which the image of God is understood in terms of certain attributes or endowments that humans possess. Foremost among them has been reason or our rational nature, the will or our voluntary nature, and our moral nature. The other view, which I am espousing and which can be characterized as "relational," goes back to Augustine and Luther. It lifts up our creaturely relation to God as the expression of the divine image in human nature. It involves our capacity to know God and to relate to God as God's human counterpart. Rather than being created "after their kind," as with other species in the Genesis account, human beings are created in the image and likeness of God.[14] This peculiar relationship between God and human beings opens the possibility of faith and trust in God as the realization of our humanity as creatures dependent upon their Creator. Rather than identifying a particular faculty or attribute as the mark of the image of God, essential as it may be to the fullness of our humanity, a definition that captures the meaning of the *imago dei* for human identity requires a far more encompassing concept.[15] For us as creatures, the fundamental reality of our existence is our relation to the Creator and to our fellow humans, bound together in our common humanity.

Our relational character means that, by nature, we are also historical beings with a past, present, and future. This captures Jürgen Moltmann's point, cited earlier in this section, in contrasting the concepts of individual and person: As individuals, we have no history but stand in isolation apart from relationships. As humans, we *become* the persons we are because of and as a result of our being in relationship. Thus, our rational and moral lives emerge and are made possible in our being related to others, expressed in the notion of personhood. Relationships also create the possibility of community as the goal and most exalted expression of life together, which means that our understanding of human nature has profound ethical implications. If by nature we are destined for community, then we are challenged to live out our lives in ways that further and support community. Whether in the context of family, church, voluntary associations, professional life, politics, or the world of commerce and business, the human obligation is to act in ways that serve the neighbor and the larger good of community. The distinctive nature of humanity brings an ethic of cooperation rather than domination, the lifting up of communitarian goals rather than the exercise of unilateral power.

This understanding of human nature bestows a divine purpose and destiny on each individual who enters the world, without regard to whether one possesses all of those faculties that we commonly identify with being human. God's relation to the person, quite apart from any abnormality or disability displayed by the person, establishes his or her identity as a child of God. A theological conviction of this kind, rooted in faith, also relativizes every other distinction we might make concerning human identity. We tend to identify people according to their parentage, their social, economic, or political status, their professional achievements, their ethnic heritage, and so on, but all of these distinctions are overruled by the one fundamental truth: all people are children of God, created for community with one another and with God, the source of their being. This means, further, that in the most fundamental sense, all people are equals, a fact that has momentous consequences for issues of political and economic justice. We are not all the same in terms of what we bring to the societal table; the differences between us are vast in regard to creativity, achievement, and contributions we make to the common good of society. But all of us command a basic respect and a claim to fundamental rights in virtue of who we are as human beings and the brute fact of our physical presence in society. Given the reality of sin and the divisiveness it creates, respect for every individual is always an ideal to be pursued more than a reality that is achieved, but the Christian understanding of who we are gives particular impetus to realizing the ideal.

Understanding the *imago dei* in terms of our relationship to God and fellow humans conveys a particularly important truth concerning our biological selves. It means that our bodily presence is essential to who we are; the body is not simply an outer garment that clothes the real self, but it constitutes the psychosomatic being that we are. A relational view of our humanity can never retreat to a Platonic notion of the soul in contrast to our bodily nature. With a relational view, we are better prepared to recognize our embeddedness in the world of nature from which we have emerged and in which we continue to exist as *Homo sapiens*. This fact is a reminder that humans are related not only to each other but also to our natural environment. The interdependence that characterizes relationships must include our relation to and dependence upon the world of nature. The support provided by that world is indispensable to our survival and well-being, a fact that commands our respect for and care of the natural environment. Paul's reference to all of creation, including ourselves, "groaning in labor pains" (Rom. 8:22-23) reflects our deep connection with all of creation and the fact that human destiny cannot be divorced from the larger world in which that destiny plays out.[16]

It is significant that the importance of relationships is recognized by scholars in the field of biological anthropology. Barbara J. King, anthropologist at the College of William and Mary, maintains in her book *Evolving God* that the emotions and mutuality involved in personal relationships are central to defining the nature of our humanity as religious beings. She places this thesis within the context of biological evolution, referring to her extensive research of the ape family, in which she finds evidence of relationships involving empathy and meaning-making activity. She argues that the beginnings of this emotional life are to be found in humanity's prehistoric ancestry, referring to such archaeological finds as burial sites where symbolic representations have been found that suggest the beginnings of the religious imagination.

A cardinal concept at which King arrives in capturing the nature of personal relationships is "belongingness," an experience that she believes is at the basis of religious life:

> And here we come to the bottom line: Hominids turned to the sacred realm because they evolved to relate in deeply emotional ways with their social partners, because the resulting mutuality engendered its own creativity and generated increasingly nuanced expressions of belongingness over time, and because the human brain evolved to allow an extension of this belongingness beyond the here and now. All of these things were necessary for the origins of the human religious imagination.[17]

King thus unites human relationships with our relation to God as our emotional experience has moved in an ever-widening circle, seeking a power greater than ourselves. Placing the root of religion in the emotional life, she notes the development of that life in the human stage with the generating of ritual and distinctive beliefs. A noteworthy and particularly welcome feature of King's approach is her focus on interpersonal relationships in addressing the phenomenon of religion, rather than focusing on the substratum of genes and neurons, which is often featured in recent attempts to "explain" religion. She acknowledges the methodological challenge of investigating an intangible concept like "belongingness" in prehistoric times; evidences of the emotional life are not typically fossilized. But her research leads her to assert that "everything we know about primates and prehistory" lends credence to the notion that the necessary emotional connections were there.[18]

## Biological Evolution and Human Nature

In forging a Christian understanding of human nature, we've noted the importance of a proper understanding of the Genesis story. That understanding frees the Christian to consider scientific accounts of human origins on their own merits, according to the evidence gathered through scientific investigations. There is little doubt within the scientific establishment (including most Christians who are scientists) that biological evolution is a fruitful theory that is indispensable in understanding how forms of life came into being. Evolutionary theory does not mean that all mystery has been removed concerning *who* the human being is, but it does help us understand *what* the human being is in relation to the rest of the biological world. Many scientific disciplines contribute toward this understanding, but in recent times, advances in genetics and molecular biology have been particularly significant in assessing the place of *Homo sapiens* within the animal kingdom. These developments have contributed substantially to a reunderstanding of Darwin's evolutionary theory. What emerged in the twentieth century was a new synthesis of genetics and microbiology, commonly called "neo-Darwinism" as a way of indicating an altered or more complete version of Darwin's original theory.

An important aspect of the genetic contribution to evolutionary theory is the light it has shed on the question "Who is our closest living relative?" Comparing humans with the great apes (including the orangutan, gorilla, chimpanzee, and bonobo) on the basis of anatomy and behavior leaves the impression that apes are much more similar to each other than to humans; they are much hairier, their arms are longer than their legs, they walk on four rather than two limbs, their brains are smaller, and their hairy faces, with large and projecting canine teeth, are quite different from the human face. While they can be taught the rudiments of sign language, their abilities to think and understand are markedly limited compared with those of humans. (While this is true, current research with chimpanzees indicates that their capacity to perform mental activities is greater than previously thought.) These larger apes together with humans constitute the five hominoid species, indicating our relatedness, but scientists since the eighteenth century have placed humans in a different zoological family: we are *hominids*, while the great apes are *pongids*. Thus, our difference is recognized within the larger family of primates.

While these observations seem reasonable enough, the findings in genetics actually suggest a different point of view. Investigations going back to the 1960s in comparative biochemistry at the molecular level reveal that, genetically and biochemically, humans and chimpanzees are more closely related than either of them is to the rhesus monkey, and that humans and African apes are more closely related to each other than either of them is to the orangutan. These conclusions have been confirmed more recently with the comparison of DNA sequences, now the ultimate mode of genetic analysis. For example, by examining amino acid sequences of one of the protein chains that makes up hemoglobin (the molecule that carries oxygen), we discover that humans and chimpanzees have all the same amino acids for this molecule, while gorillas share all but one. Another study in 1975 showed that humans and chimpanzees share over 98 percent of their DNA, unmistakable evidence that they have evolved from a common ancestor. (It is interesting to note, however, that genetics doesn't help us understand how such genetic similarity can be found in creatures whose morphology, or physical appearance, can be so different from ours.) It is not surprising that scientists are debating how to classify humans, with some favoring a system that recognizes our relatedness to the African apes, while others prefer a system that recognizes our differences.[19] Within the context of scientific classification, it is another indication, you might say, of the two-sided understanding that human identity inherently raises.

There is no reason for Christians to react defensively to these evidences of our biological continuity with the lower primates. We are so used to stressing our uniqueness as human beings that any reminder of our connectedness with the animal world is often regarded as a threat.

This way of thinking reflects the genetic fallacy, where we identify our origin with our nature; this fallacy fails to recognize the emergent character of human nature, where we *become* who we are. There is certainly enough evidence of our uniqueness as human beings to dispel any reason for alarm in recognizing our biological origin and our embeddedness in the animal world. That uniqueness begins with our physical existence, where scientists point out the significant differences in body structure and anatomy between humans and other primates; these differences in turn make possible the more profound differences that distinguish us from the rest of the animal kingdom. For example, among the vertebrates, we are the only species holding an erect posture and moving in a bipedal gait, and our arms, hands, and thumbs are arranged so as to enable precise manipulation, features that make possible our command of the environment. Most importantly, our vocal tract, possessing a longer pharynx than that of our ancestors, makes possible the phenomenon of speech, which is essential to the development of language, commonly acknowledged as the distinguishing feature of our humanity.[20]

The most significant difference between humans and other animals is found in the brain. Humans have the largest brain among primates, with a weight in the adult male of approximately three pounds, compared with roughly one pound in the gorilla and slightly less than that in the chimpanzee. Related to this is the fact that in the average mammal, about 3 percent of the blood pumped by its heart services the brain; in humans, it is close to 16 percent. Neuropsychologists tell us that brain size relative to body weight increased dramatically with the emergence of humans. In addition, the human cerebral cortex, where cognitive processes take place, is disproportionately larger in relation to the rest of the brain than is the case with apes—roughly three times the size it would be in other primates of equal size.

But weight and size alone are not the only distinctive features (the brains of whales and elephants are larger than those of humans). One also finds much greater complexity in the human brain, with a degree of specialization that is unique, particularly cerebral asymmetries and areas in the neocortex associated with speech. As the number of neurons (nerve cells) in a nervous system increases, so does the complexity of an animal's behavioral responses. Amazingly, the human brain contains more than ten billion neurons, extending over sixty thousand miles, with each neuron making hundreds, even thousands, of links with others. An immense number of nerve fibers move from the brain through the spinal cord, in contact with some billion sensory units from which they receive electrical signals from all parts of the body. It is this marvelous complexity and specialization of the brain and nervous system—by far the most complex structure in the universe—that literally opens up the possibility of human consciousness and human culture.

Physicists speak of "phase transitions" where the circumstances give rise to something that is distinctively new. For example, in the transition from ice to water or from water to steam, elements that remain the same are dramatically changed; something quite different emerges. Biologists use this notion of a phase change in the context of biological evolution, where a major increase in the capacity of abilities at one level results in a new level of complexity. The concept is used to account for the radically new character of the emerging brain in the human species. With the emergence of this remarkable organ, evolving over hundreds of thousands of years, we see the entry of those qualities distinctive to the human being as a counterpart to the Creator: the attributes of sensation and perception, of thought and cognition, of emotion and feeling, of consciousness and self-awareness, of moral and religious experience. This is not to say that other primates fail to give evidence of at least some of these characteristics—the continuity with other primates is still there—but the range and depth of these attributes in human beings are stunningly new. While a rudimentary consciousness can be recognized in some of the higher animals, human self-consciousness is a further development that has brought a corresponding awareness of the presence of God and the distinctive world of human relationships that together have set us apart among all creatures of the world.

## Reconceptualizing the Soul

Many Christians would question whether the preceding discussion, limited as it is to human anatomy and genetics, can begin to do justice to the essential nature and uniqueness of the human being. They would claim that we cannot talk about that uniqueness without talking about the soul. It is indeed true that, throughout Christian history, a dualistic understanding of human beings has prevailed: the concept of the soul in contrast to the body has literally defined the essence and uniqueness of the human being. Understandably, this fact generated much of the resistance to Darwin's theory. The Roman Catholic anatomist George Jackson Mivart (1827–1900) argued that evolution could be seen as a natural explanation for the development of the human body but could not explain the human soul. The soul had to be a divine creation, befitting its uniqueness as a spiritual entity. It took some time for this compromise position to be accepted by the church hierarchy (Mivart himself was excommunicated), but it eventually became the Roman Catholic position on this issue. Pope John Paul II addressed the topic in his 1996 annual address to the Pontifical Academy of the Sciences, where he essentially recognized biological evolution as scientific fact but limited it to the physical nature of the human being.[21]

When one considers the biblical witness concerning the soul, however, the consensus among biblical scholars is that the Hebrew Scriptures (the Christian Old Testament) present quite clearly a holistic or unified view of human nature, in contrast to a dualistic view.[22] The story of creation is particularly significant here: the "breath of life" endowed by God (Gen. 2:7) makes a living being with an animated or spirited body, rather than God creating a soul and giving it a temporal home by placing it in the body. While there are Hebrew words that we translate as "soul" (*nephesh*) and "spirit" (*ruach*, also translated as "breath"), in the Hebrew mind, they do not refer to distinct entities that could exist outside of the body. They are functional words that refer to the whole person and describe human activities such as thinking and feeling, often understood as coming from the organ of the heart. This holistic way of discourse characterizes Hebrew in contrast to Greek thinking. The human being is ontologically one, not two, with inner and outer dimensions captured by such terms as *soul* and *body*.

The New Testament reveals aspects of Greek thinking in its language, but one can hardly argue that it conveys a dualistic view of the human being. Particularly in the letters of the apostle Paul, there are references to the spiritual life in which words such as *psyche* ("soul" or inner life or being) and *pneuma* ("spirit") are used, and this language has been interpreted in ways that encourage the notion of a spiritual essence of the human that is real and eternal in contrast to the body. Given the pervasiveness of Greek influence in the developing theology of the early church, this development is not surprising. Among the early church fathers, the dominant influence was the Greek philosopher Plato, who held to a dualism of body and soul, with the latter being the eternal essence of the human being. The body belongs to the material world marked by mortality, a shadow world that lacks the reality of spirit.

The most threatening heresy in the early centuries of the church was Gnosticism, which placed the spiritual world in sharp contrast to the material world, as in the contrast between good and evil. Being both body and soul, human beings are caught in the middle of this conflict; the religious and moral life is pursued by nurturing the spiritual life and battling the temptations rooted in our bodily existence. This kind of thinking was pervasive throughout the ancient world, including the Christian community; it served as a paradigm for understanding life's journey and the moral challenges it raised. During the twentieth century, which witnessed a renaissance in biblical studies, Protestant scholars generally came to the conclusion that the New Testament does not convey the kind of dualism that took hold in the ancient church. The belief in the resurrection of the dead defines the position of the New Testament, revealing a clear alternative to the notion of a disembodied soul as the identifying and immortal part of the human being. The future life is marked by resurrection and transformation, not the departure of the soul from the body. Paul's discussion of the resurrection in 1 Corinthians 15 places our future solely in the transforming act of God rather than any capacity within ourselves—such as an eternal soul—that would guarantee our immortality.

In light of these reflections, many Christians would ask all the more urgently, and perhaps with a measure of exasperation, "What about the soul?" My intent is not to dispense with the word (as though that were possible), but to clarify its meaning and proper usage within the Christian community. We often use the word *soul* in a figurative sense to refer to the essence of a person, the "real me." That usage serves a good purpose as long as the word retains its figurative character. To put it differently, *soul* should be recognized as a *functional* word; we are "soul-like," but we do not "have" a soul. It expresses the inner life of humans that marks their distinctive existence as spiritual beings, attuned to transcendence and sensitive to questions of ultimate meaning and purpose. Augustine's comment in his *Confessions* concerning a human "restlessness" that finds its rest in God is a particularly apt expression of our spiritual nature. The word *soul* is most often used in reference to religious experience, but it functions within a wide enough range of human experience to make it inherently ambiguous. It can be understood conceptually as the life principle or core of one's being (Aristotle's view, in which the soul as the "form" of the body expresses its purpose, or *telos*), without introducing the notion of a separate metaphysical entity that exists apart from the body (Plato's view). For the person of faith, the word *soul* conveys our capacity to stand in relationship to God as well as to our fellow human beings, without whom it would be impossible to claim and express our human identity.

Some language analysis may be helpful in making my point that the word *soul* is to be understood in a functional sense. Because it serves as a noun (which by definition denotes a person, place, or thing), *soul* is understood as denoting a thing or entity. Language can play tricks on us this way, where we reify ("thingify") a concept rather than addressing its experiential meaning. When we do the latter, we find it more appropriate simply to speak of ourselves as spiritual beings created in God's image, with the word *soul* capturing that reality rather than introducing an entity that skews Christian anthropology in a dualistic direction. The point is that to affirm our nature as spiritual beings and creatures of God does not require the existence of a soul. To recognize this also spares one from the thorny problem of having to locate the soul somewhere within the body. Plato placed it in the "marrow" of the head, presumably the brain. Moschion, a renowned Greek physician of the second century, maintained that the soul floats throughout the whole body. The philosopher René Descartes (1596–1650), who has been most influential in shaping the contemporary dualistic understanding, placed the soul in the pineal gland at the base of the brain. Given the obscure nature of this gland at the time, it was a fairly persuasive conclusion. Less well known is the conclusion of the eighteenth-century French surgeon Gigot de la Peyronie, who claimed on the basis of some rather bizarre experiments that the seat of the soul must be the corpus callosum, deep within the brain.

Among other things, we avoid such attempts at location when we recognize that to speak of the soul is simply to recognize our spiritual nature: As creatures of God, created in God's image, we respond in awe to the mystery of God and grapple with ultimate kinds of questions concerning our human nature and identity. As creatures of God, we live by faith, recognizing spiritual or depth dimensions to human experience that aren't adequately captured by the language and concepts of the sciences. Human consciousness enables us to see ourselves not only as embodied and physically identified beings, but also as capable of self-transcendence and self-reflection, raising the kinds of questions we are considering here about human identity. A functional understanding of the soul applies also to the concept of the mind, which is not an entity apart from the body but a descriptive term that refers to human consciousness and the cerebral activities we call thinking, reasoning, and reflecting. We will continue to use words like *soul* and *mind* as nouns because doing so is a shorthand way of referring to the realities they represent, but that practice shouldn't seduce us into thinking that they denote existing entities.

In the minds of most Christians, perhaps, the concept of the soul is particularly related to human destiny and life beyond the grave. In popular religion, the soul seems to be required in order to affirm that we shall live beyond death; by definition, it is not affected by the mortality of the body. From the perspective of a more deeply rooted biblical position, as we have noted, this view is contradicted by the good news that our destiny lies in the hands of God, who is sovereign over both life and death. There is no reference whatsoever to an "immortal soul" in the New Testament. Its witness places both Jesus' destiny and our own squarely in God with the teaching of the resurrection of the dead. Thus, from a biblical point of view, our destiny lies in the transformative power of God, who can make all things new. We can say that any reference to the mystery of an afterlife is an expression of faith in God as Lord over both our present and our future.

## Concluding Thoughts

Our discussion of human nature in Christian perspective has affirmed the complementarity of science and religion, in contrast to notions of conflict and antagonism. This concept has been helpful in recent years in assisting the faith community to effectively relate the concerns of science and religious faith, but it can also be misunderstood. Its value is that it recognizes the essential difference between religion and science in the kinds of interests, goals, and purposes that each brings to the subject of human nature, the kinds of questions that each consequently raises, and the insights that are elicited. But these differences are misunderstood if they lead one to hermetically seal science from religion or religion from science, preventing the possibility of fruitful dialogue. Their different methodologies do not logically exclude theology from considering the implications of scientific investigation for the larger questions of meaning and purpose that theology wants to explore. Nor do those differences exclude the sciences from investigating those theological claims that by their nature are subject to scientific investigation. Because both science and theology are interested in the question of human nature, they necessarily meet at that point and are challenged to recognize what they can learn from the other.

A recent initiative to introduce the concept of "consonance" in place of "complementarity" in describing the relation of theology and the natural sciences reflects the desire to affirm and emphasize the unity of truth and the necessary harmony of science and religion. This view argues that complementarity (often referred to as the "two-language" view) prevents communication between science and religion because it consigns each to a wholly different realm of language and conceptualities.[23] I've noted this danger but still believe that it is necessary to recognize the differing mind-set and consequent difference in focus and interest in each of these disciplines. Truth is indeed a unity, but complementarity is a concept that recognizes this fact at the same time that it respects differing approaches to the truth. The distinctive faith of the Christian theologian brings the world of nature into the realm of creation and a creator God, an orientation that scientists—whatever religious faith they might have—cannot allow to influence the empirical assumptions that govern the nature of their work. Any dialogue between science and theology moves beyond those assumptions to a secondary level, where explicitly philosophical and theological inferences are drawn from scientific investigation. This "meta-level" of discourse is where the opportunity for dialogue and cross-fertilization of ideas can take place. It involves recognition of the distinctive character of each discipline as well as their legitimate interest in a common subject matter and the insights that each can bring to it.

Christians today as never before are challenged to inform themselves about evolutionary biology, to understand its essential role in the work of the life sciences, and to move beyond the assumption that it must be a mortal threat to their faith. The biblical witness recognizes our embeddedness in the world of nature and, unlike much of the tradition in Christian anthropology, does not seek to escape it or deny it. The dualistic tradition that still holds sway in the church encourages a false denial of our biological roots or, at the very least, an attempt to ignore what we have learned about human origins. The tragedy of this situation is that people of faith deny their own calling when they fail to be truthful with themselves concerning the results of responsible scholarship. They need to understand that biblical faith allows us to affirm our uniqueness both as children of God and as children of nature.

In speaking of the complementarity of science and Christian faith, we can also recognize the complementarity of body and soul in our understanding of human nature. Biological evolution can help us to understand that these two concepts are no longer to be regarded as ontological opposites and exclusive to each other. We can now recognize that biological life gives rise to the spiritual life, serving as a foundation that enables the human capacity for transcendence and what we call the image of God. The incredible complexity of the brain gives rise to something new and uniquely human, enabling the life of relationships that shape our personhood and self-understanding. Rather than reducing our spiritual life to its biological foundation—an effort that is alive and well in what we call scientific materialism or scientific naturalism—we can recognize its reality and integrity in defining who we are as spirited creatures. We are now in a position as Christians to recognize and embrace both matter and spirit, the bodily and the spiritual life, as a psychosomatic, interdependent unity. The body, in response to its environment, gives rise to the life of the spirit, and that spirit-life both directs and fulfills our existence in the world.

CHAPTER 2

# Human Nature and Biological Reductionism

An obvious reason for the church's attraction to dualistic thinking, in which an eternal soul is posited in an earthly body, is that Christians think it is the only way to avoid a purely physical or materialistic view of the human being. Thus, a belief in the existence of the soul appears as the hallmark of a Christian anthropology or of any religious understanding of human nature. Since the nature of human beings is a continuing issue for the biological sciences, it is not surprising that religious views often come under scientific appraisal. In modern times, there has been no lack of scientists who have questioned and repudiated the dualism common to religious views. Is there space for a meeting of minds between theologians and scientists in their understanding of human nature? As theologians incorporate findings from evolutionary biology and reconceptualize their understanding of the soul in order to maintain a genuinely holistic view of the human being, a more serious attempt can be made to dialogue with those who engage the subject from a scientific point of view. Indeed, the possibility of finding common ground between theologians and scientists is more promising today than ever before.

Other factors also play a role in this convergence. In a postmodern world that stresses the contextualization of truth, and where relativism seems to be running rampant, one of the casualties has been the notion of a universal human nature. The natural sciences stand in contrast to this kind of thinking and could well be an ally with those concerned to form a theological anthropology. Theologians clearly operate with a "big picture," seeing the human story in light of God's creation and understanding human nature in universal terms. Evolutionary biology also projects a big picture, bringing human and natural history together in one unified history and making a universal human nature a meaningful concept. The challenge for theologians is to find natural scientists with whom they can work in fashioning a vision of human nature that draws on both theological and scientific resources.[1]

Of course, scientists are far from speaking with one voice on the subject of human nature. There have always been those who espouse a materialist philosophy on the basis of their understanding of the implications of scientific investigations; they identify science with a worldview that stands in opposition to what Christians believe. They also tend to identify Christian belief with the positions of fundamentalist Christians, who are easy targets for those seeking to link religion with obscurantism. They are, you might say, knights of the Enlightenment, still fighting the irrationalities they identify with religion. Because some of these scientists have achieved national acclaim through their writings and have exercised considerable influence far beyond scientific circles—Edward O. Wilson and Richard Dawkins are two prominent examples—it is important to address their arguments here. They are among those on the scientific side who would find little promise in efforts to fashion a complementary relationship between science and theology.

## Scientific Materialism

One of the most eloquent voices among these "scientific philosophers" is that of Edward O. Wilson. A two-time Pulitzer Prize winner and holder of the National Medal of Science among many other distinguished awards, Wilson has made his reputation as a scientist in the field of insect life, or entomology, but his interests run far beyond his discipline.

Though calling himself a "scientific humanist," Wilson can appropriately be characterized as an evangelist for scientific materialism, which he ardently advocates as a worldview that can rescue humanity from all the false and futile beliefs that until now have claimed its allegiance. In his book *On Human Nature*, published in 1978, Wilson recognizes three major myths that at that time were governing people's lives and creating considerable political and intellectual strife: Marxism, traditional religion, and scientific materialism. With Marxism in decline, he proposes scientific materialism as the one substantive alternative to religious belief:

> Make no mistake about the power of scientific materialism. It presents the mind with an alternative mythology that until now has always, point for point in zones of conflict, defeated traditional religion. . . . Every part of existence is considered to be obedient to physical laws requiring no external control. . . . We have come to the crucial stage in the history of biology when religion itself is subject to the explanations of the natural sciences. . . . The final decisive edge enjoyed by scientific naturalism will come from its capacity to explain traditional religion, its chief competitor, as a wholly material phenomenon.[2]

This statement of Wilson is a philosophical assertion based on a reductionist thesis, which maintains that the final verdict concerning human nature is to be found at the micro level of biochemical reactions that occur in the body and most importantly in the brain. This means that our subjective experience, including our mental life and self-consciousness, can be reduced to and therefore explained and defined by the physical activity that takes place at the molecular level. The human being as a thinking, imagining, willing, and emotive subject relating to other human subjects, cultural life, and the global environment is ultimately reduced to what goes on in biochemical reactions at the molecular level. Complexity that challenges our comprehension receives a rather facile explanation by use of a "bottom-up" methodology that reduces complexity to the relative simplicity of physicochemical activity in the brain. The seductive appeal of this kind of reasoning is enhanced by the fact that the trademark of scientific investigation is a reductionist methodology; science understands the human body by reducing it to its component parts.

Thus, it is critically important that we make a clear distinction between methodological reductionism as an essential activity of science and its extension to the much broader field of philosophical understanding. When Wilson assumes that the reductionist principle provides the ultimate, definitive understanding of the total life and experience of the human being, he is transforming a scientific, methodological principle into a materialist, philosophical argument. More than this, Wilson is proposing with his concept of "sociobiology" to "reformulate the foundations of the social sciences," creating a new synthesis that would ultimately embrace all knowledge of the human being.[3] Researchers in the social sciences and the humanities, whose study of the human being involves methodologies far removed from those of the natural sciences, should narrow their focus and recognize that humans are essentially physical objects of study. This belief that the natural sciences are the one source of significant knowledge about the world, including the human being, has been characterized as "scientism." Given the determining role Wilson ascribes to the natural sciences, there is considerable irony in his claim that sociobiology should be seen as a bridge concept at the juncture of biology and psychology, creating a synthesis between them and ultimately between the two realms of the sciences and the humanities. He believes that the chasm between them, dramatized so eloquently by C. P. Snow in *The Two Cultures and the Scientific Revolution* (1959), can now finally be overcome, but only by translating psychology into biology.

Wilson concludes that the concept of the mind "will be more precisely explained as an epiphenomenon of the neuronal machinery of the brain."[4] He assumes that if we no longer regard the mind as a spiritual entity, then a materialist view is logically necessary, and human nature itself can be described completely and exclusively in empirical terms. It is true that when we reject the traditional dualism of mind and body, we recognize at the same time the need and legitimacy of utilizing the so-called brain sciences—the research of neurobiologists and cognitive psychologists—in addressing the stream of human experience, both conscious and subconscious. The avenues to understanding that stream obviously include empirical investigations of the neurons, neurotransmitters, and hormones that are indispensable to it. But acknowledging this point hardly requires the adoption of philosophical materialism.

With the development of highly sophisticated technology, research done with localized brain damage has contributed immensely to our understanding of the functions performed by different parts of the brain. Wilson makes particular point of the fact that all we know from this kind of brain research gives no evidence of there being an organizing center in the brain; there is no "executive ego" that is monitoring neural processes in the various parts of the brain that might indicate a mind or self at work.[5] On the contrary, the mind is "the brain at work." For the Christian who rejects a dualist view of mind/body, it appears quaint to look for evidence of a mind or soul at work in the brain; it reminds one of Soviet Premier Nikita Khrushchev's remark that God was nowhere to be seen on the first flight into outer space. There is, in fact, little reason to question Wilson's discussion of the mind as "the brain at work." One can recognize that the neural activity going on in the brain is essential to the mental activity that forms human consciousness without thereby denying what we want to affirm with the concept of mind. As I noted in chapter 1, and contrary to Wilson's view, the mind should be understood as a functional word rather than an entity—a verb rather than a noun. It is a concept that stands for mental activity, our thinking and reasoning and the sense of our subjective self that is inherent to such activity. This functional understanding of the mind does not appear to register with sociobiologists, who see only two alternatives: either the mind is reduced to the operations of the brain, or it is a spiritual entity that requires a dualistic view of the human being. They then confidently proceed to repudiate the latter view on the basis of scientific reasoning.

In more recent years, Wilson has elaborated on his quest for a unified theory of knowledge that closes the gap between the sciences and humanities. He uses the word *consilience* to express this unification of knowledge that will provide for the first time a common groundwork of explanation for all the phenomena we encounter in the world. This "common groundwork," once again, reflects a reductionist thesis; consilience holds "that nature is organized by simple universal laws of physics to which all other laws and principles can eventually be reduced."[6]

No matter how complex, all of life, including the mental and emotional life of human beings, finds its ultimate expression in the language of biology and genetics; the language of the natural sciences gives us the most promising avenue toward the universal understanding we seek. Wilson sees himself in the train of Enlightenment philosophers but with a critical difference: thanks to neo-Darwinism, we are now equipped to actually achieve the unity and coherence of thought and understanding that eluded the eighteenth-century philosophers. The basic questions concerning human nature—Who are we? Where have we come from? What is our destiny?—can now receive definitive answers based on scientific evidence.

While Wilson maintains a materialist viewpoint throughout, one can detect some modifications in his stance between *On Human Nature* (1978) and *Consilience* (1998). Any reference to God in the former work is consistently disparaged, but he allows for a deistic stance in the latter book (he has more recently described himself as a "provisional deist"), where a God who creates the evolutionary process is now withdrawn from that process. Wilson's attitude toward religion is actually ambivalent; he acknowledges the legitimacy of a profound drive within the human spirit to make sense out of life, to find ultimate answers concerning the meaning of things. His conclusion, to the consternation of many of his fellow scientists, is to treat science as a new religion that now provides the answers we have been seeking. "Could Holy Writ be just the first literate attempt to explain the universe and make ourselves significant within it? Perhaps science is a continuation on new and better-tested ground to attain the same end. If so, then in that sense science is religion liberated and writ large."[7] Clearly, Wilson is a thinker who wants to arrive at the "big picture." To do so, he appropriates the universal claims befitting religious faith, but it leads to an ironic picture. The natural sciences offer no message of meaning and hope that can compare with the message of religious faiths. What meaning can one glean from biology, for example, other than the determination to survive? Such an answer avoids the risk involved in taking the "leap of faith" of which Christians speak, but at the expense of losing the fulfillment found in religious and ethical commitment that creatures reflecting the image of God quite naturally seek.

Another feature worth noting in Wilson's work is the increased attention he gives to the environment in his understanding of human behavior. In *Consilience*, the role of culture becomes more prominent as Wilson now speaks of "gene-culture coevolution" in the shaping of human nature, and while genetics keeps culture on a firm leash, the relation between them contains some flexibility. The more rapid the cultural change, the "looser" becomes that connection as humans adapt to their environment "without correspondingly precise genetic prescription. In this respect human beings differ fundamentally from all other animal species."[8] But Wilson's hedging hardly constitutes a meaningful change in his bottom-up approach. He sees culture as operating according to laws of natural selection and not independently of biological evolution; there is no real acknowledgment of culture as a source of genesis in understanding human behavior. The end result of his materialist view is a biological-chemical explanation of the whole realm of spiritual life and the distinctive experiences of purpose and intentionality that mark human existence.

## The Response of Intelligent Design

My discussion of scientific materialism has focused particularly on the mind/body problem within the context of biological evolution. Materialists like Wilson understand the process of natural selection that accounts for biological evolution in thoroughly materialist terms, leaving no room for nonphysical categories in understanding the human being. Before bringing a theological critique to this view of humanity, it will be helpful to note some theological responses that create more problems than they resolve. Two such responses, based on the assumption that Darwinian evolution is an atheistic explanation of the evolutionary process, are Intelligent Design (ID) and its cousin, scientific creationism.[9]

The theory of natural selection, which is Darwin's distinctive contribution to the *how* of biological evolution, does not recognize any direction or design in the process of evolution. Natural selection appears to be random rather than demonstrating an overarching purpose or inevitability, a conclusion that is shared among the vast majority of biologists today. ID advocates would refute this claim by arguing that, on the basis of a purely empirical, scientific reading of the evidence, one must conclude that intelligence and design are quite evident in evolution. The problem with this claim is that scientific disciplines do not allow any reference to design, because the concept immediately implies a Designer, or God, which in turn introduces a supernatural explanation where only natural (scientific) explanations are acceptable. One destroys the working assumptions critical to scientific investigation if one introduces the notion of God as an explanatory factor in understanding the phenomena of the natural world. To emphasize design also raises problems in light of the fact that there are many anomalies in the natural world that do not fit very well with the notion of an omniscient Designer who presumably makes no mistakes.

ID advocates will deny any reference to God as such, but the implications of their language clearly move beyond science to theology. Their arguments are more sophisticated than those of the creationists, who freely acknowledge a religious basis for their point of view; the Bible's account of creation stands behind their repudiation of biological evolution. ID proponents argue instead that natural selection is simply an inadequate explanation for what we observe in the biological world. A central tenet of ID proponents is "irreducible complexity," where they claim that the presence of multiple parts in highly complex organs, such as the eye, cannot be explained or accounted for on the basis of the step-by-step process of evolution that is presumed by Darwin's theory. This argument has been repudiated by scientists, but the particular point to be made here is that making design a "scientific" conclusion oversteps a critical boundary and results in confusing the nature of both science and religion.

People of faith readily echo the words of the psalmist:

> When I look at your heavens, the work of your fingers,
> > the moon and the stars that you have established;
> what are human beings that you are mindful of them,
> > mortals that you care for them?
> Yet you have made them a little lower than God,
> > and crowned them with glory and honor. (Ps. 8:3-5)

This picturesque language reveals the attitude of faith, overwhelmed by the awesome mystery of nature and humanity and ascribing to them a meaning and a status that are foreign to scientific understanding. We have here the juxtaposition of *mythos* and *logos*, the religious and scientific temperament that every thoughtful person must negotiate within his or her own understanding. While the sentiments of the psalmist certainly invite the notion of design, it is a concept that can hardly be integrated with a scientific discipline. Evolutionary biologists speak of "adaptation," which expresses the process of natural selection in which organisms evolve in the struggle for existence and survival. Quite obviously, it is a process that has yielded tremendous complexity and diversity over a vast number of years and in incremental stages. People of faith see it as an intelligible process that at least suggests a divine Intelligence, but they cannot claim any kind of scientific proof for that claim. There is complementarity here between scientific and theological viewpoints; they can live together, but only as they respect the appropriateness of the methodology that each brings to the understanding of *Homo sapiens*. Neither view is in a position simply to refute the other.

Because ID advocates regard the reigning interpretation of biological evolution as the expression of an atheistic, materialist philosophy, it is understandable that their response is at the same level of discourse—a philosophical/theological response that claims scientific validity on the basis of empirical data as they interpret it. As such, I believe ID can best be understood as a contemporary example of natural theology, a venerable but also controversial tradition in the history of philosophy and of Christian thought. Notions of design and purpose evident in the world and universe have led philosophers and theologians from the Middle Ages if not ancient times to claim the necessity of a divine being as the source of it all. William Paley, in his book *Natural Theology* (1802), offered an appealing analogy in which the world is likened to a watch: the only way to account for the watch is to infer the existence of a watchmaker. Similarly, ID advocates see in the complexity of the human being the necessity of a designer but refrain from referring to a divine designer. We can conclude that the arguments of both Wilson and ID advocates mix philosophical or theological assumptions with scientific reasoning in ways that invalidate their conclusions. Scientific investigation does not establish a materialist worldview any more than it proves a divine designer. The thesis that theology (or philosophy) and science are complementary to each other seeks to avoid this confusion by recognizing that each brings its distinctive epistemology (ways of knowing) and methodology to the same subject, each creating its own context of meaning.

Many scientists and theologians working at the junctures of science and theology—including some whose education has included extensive study in both theology and the natural sciences—recognize this truth and offer a more careful, nuanced approach in relating the two areas. John Polkinghorne, internationally recognized theoretical physicist and canon theologian in the Anglican Church, makes the point that, in relation to nature, science is a first-order activity that deals directly with the physical world, while theology is a second-order activity that seeks to integrate the results of first-order investigations into a metaphysical or theological understanding of the world. These two different activities are clearly not symmetrical to each other but can be and should be seen as complementary.[10] As to the actual reading of scientific evidence, ID proponents tend to bolster their case by exaggerating the *random* character of genetic mutation and the consequent inadequacy of Darwinism to account for the emergence of such a complicated organism as the human being. Actually, Darwin himself does not use the term *random* in *The Origin of Species*. The term is used by evolutionary biologists to make the point that the occurrence of mutations is independent of any useful purpose they might have, but these scientists would also acknowledge that mutations can become useful within the process of natural selection.[11] Polkinghorne suggests that greater insight into that process might lead in the direction of positing holistic laws of nature "that encourage the formation of certain kinds of pattern and inhibit the formation of others," thus assisting the direction toward fruitful change that is evident in the evolutionary process.[12] The *combination* of law and chance would seem to best explain what is happening in natural selection.

The late Arthur Peacocke, eminent biochemist and later priest and canon in the Church of England, also brings a responsible critique to various understandings of natural selection. He notes that the emphasis on "survival of the fittest" (a phrase widely used by Thomas Huxley and subsequently adopted by Darwin) unfortunately encourages an exclusively "red in tooth and claw" perception of evolution. Such factors as better integration with the ecological environment, better care of the young, and more cooperative social organization also are important to survival.[13] As with Polkinghorne, Peacocke refers to the interplay between chance and law in natural selection, seeing the original mutational events in the DNA as random with respect to the future of the organism, but the "biological niche" in which the organism exists favoring "in a law-like way" those changes in the DNA that enable it to produce and rear more progeny. Mutation occurs in random fashion at the micro level, but rather than proving the irrationality of the universe, it opens up all the potentialities of living matter. Given the structures in which life develops, the end result is creative advance rather than uncontrollable occurrence. Both chance and inevitability are built into the process, making possible an ordered universe that is capable of developing new modes of existence from within itself.[14] This process offers no *proof* of God, but it certainly invites a sense of awe and meaningfulness for the person of religious faith. Polkinghorne and Peacocke avoid making theological claims under the guise of science, respecting the distinctive realm of each. At the same time, they are able to bring constructive, alternative proposals to a scientific debate, inspired by their scientific knowledge as well as their theistic convictions.[15]

## A Critique of Scientific Materialism

If we reject a dualistic position in which soul and mind exist apart from the cellular activity of the body, how does the Christian respond to scientific materialism? One response to the attempt to reduce our mental life to physiological processes is that it involves what philosophers call a categorical mistake: two different conceptual realms are confused as one. There is a jump from the language or realm of physiology to the realm of subjective consciousness, from addressing objects in space to experiencing events in time, apparently without questioning whether that jump doesn't destroy the logic of one's deduction. In the one case, where the neural patterns of the brain are examined, we gain knowledge from a third-person perspective. In the other case, where we address our consciousness and self-awareness, we are involved subjectively and immediately in a first-person perspective. The question is how to relate these two contexts in a way that maintains the integrity of each instead of dissolving the one into the other.

This is a subject that until recently fell within the province of philosophers rather than scientists, but with the development of technology such as scanners that can track the activity of the brain, the field of cognitive neuroscience is now addressing the subject of human consciousness. Scientists disagree whether we can ever explain how our subjective experience arises from neural activity; how would we go about bridging the gap between our observation of brain activity and the experience of consciousness? Some would conclude that it is an inherently unsolvable problem because we don't even know what a solution would look like. It would literally demand the creation of a new language with concepts that transcend the current divide between the "physical" and "mental," but how would we arrive there? Others firmly believe that we can and will arrive at a satisfactory answer, but they tend to espouse positions identified with the empirical sciences. Where everyone agrees is that the brain sciences have succeeded in tracking the biochemical activity in the brain that clearly correlates with the thoughts and emotions experienced by the human subject.[16]

To illustrate, we know that the limbic lobes of the brain are the site where emotions are kindled and various psychological drives are set in motion. If one hears a sound that induces fright, the anatomy and physiology of what happens can be described as objective events: pressure waves set in motion by sound reach the inner ear, causing nerve impulses in the auditory nerve, causing further impulses that reach those regions of the brain where the sound is recognized and corresponding emotions are evoked. But does this explain the experience of fright? It would appear that we are explaining an anatomical and physiological process, but not the subjective experience itself. The proper conclusion is not to insist on the existence of a mind in order to account for the subjective experience, but to recognize that mental and emotional experiences characterize human awareness and have their own integrity. To reduce the subjective experience to the physiological description is not only a logical blunder but an assault on the richness and depth of human consciousness.

If we acknowledge that a dualistic position is not a viable alternative to a materialist view, then different language is called for in relating the bodily context to that of the mental. It is language that does not *reduce* mental life to physiology but rather recognizes our mental life as indeed *rooted* or *based* in the processes of the brain and nervous system. We are psychobiological beings whose mental life is clearly rooted in the brain without being *defined* by what goes on in the brain. Malcolm Jeeves elaborates this point of view, which he describes as "nonreductive physicalism":

> A formulation of the nonreductive physicalist view that we believe does justice to the evidence currently available would regard mental activity and correlated brain activity as inner and outer aspects of one complex set of events which together constitute conscious human agency.... According to this view, we regard mental activity as *embodied in* brain activity rather than as being *identical with* brain activity.[17]

Stating the matter a bit differently but making the same essential point, the philosopher Philip Kitcher observes that most important is the point that "the intricate neural firings moving us to act constitute wishes and intentions that accord with our self-conceptions. Molecular biology promises to dissect the self, but we need not fear that it will remove from our vision those aspects that lend special meaning to our lives."[18] The critical point in this philosophical debate is to maintain the distinctive language required by our subjective experience; it is not to be explained away or channeled into a strict system of biological cause and effect. Neither is it to be justified by positing a mind, a kind of inner sanctum beyond the reach of science. Our mental experience is more than neuronal activity but is dependent upon it.[19]

Theologians and philosophers are not the only ones who take exception to the reductionist argument. One of Wilson's more prominent antagonists was a longtime colleague at Harvard University, the late Stephen Jay Gould. A paleontologist by profession but, like Wilson, a man of many pursuits ranging well beyond his discipline, Gould saw in Wilson the perennial but ill-fated attempt to reduce all knowledge to one common denominator. The fatal flaw in his reductionist thesis, says Gould, is that all complex systems involve interactions that introduce new or emergent elements that cannot be reduced to their lower-level parts. This principle of emergence becomes increasingly important as we mount the scale of complexity. A second principle articulated by Gould is that of contingency, which marks the historical development of complex organisms and makes impossible any attempt at explanations that are totally predictable. The "accidental" reasons involved in unique historical events, with their consequent impact on organisms, cannot be explained by classical reductionism.[20] Consonant with his rejection of reductionism, Gould maintains the integrity of the humanities—and of religion in particular—as distinctive domains ("magisteria") with their own language and methods that stand in contrast to those of the sciences.[21]

Antonio Damasio is a neuroscientist whose research on the brain has led to conclusions that also stand in contrast to those of scientific materialism. Professor of neuroscience and director of the Brain and Creativity Institute at the University of Southern California, Damasio has done pioneering work in the neural systems that subserve human emotions and the cognitive life.[22] Contrary to the philosophical reductionists, Damasio sees the biology of the brain as providing the mechanisms necessary to human consciousness and self-awareness, reason and moral insight, but does not espouse a philosophical model that would explain consciousness by reducing it to biological categories. In an interview with *The Harvard Brain*, Damasio observes that any attempt to understand the relation between brain systems and complex cognition and behavior demands a comprehensive approach that encompasses everything from the molecular level to the macro world of physical and social environments. "In other words, beware of explanations that rely on data from one single level, whatever the level may be."[23] This is sound advice, not only for materialists but also for those whose understanding of mind and soul tempts them to explain the spiritual life apart from the physiology of the brain.

The attempt to explain all human action on the basis of molecular activity, which we see in scientific materialism (what we have called a bottom-up understanding), can also be challenged on the basis of our knowledge of the neuronal makeup of the brain. The biological anthropologist Barbara J. King observes that there is considerable plasticity in the human brain as it relates to the environment: "Communication between particular neurons can be strengthened by experience; learning thus changes the brain. It also appears now that entire networks of neurons—indeed, whole brain regions—may be similarly affected by experience."[24] Experiments with blind persons reveal that the brain is capable of reorganizing itself when challenged by the environment. When a blind person reads Braille, touching the bumps on the page, it is the *visual* part of the brain that responds to a new kind of task. Experiments with musicians show that their brains are highly adaptable; one study found that the auditory cortex in musicians was 130 percent larger than in nonmusicians, with the degree of increase correlated with the extent of musical training.[25] These kinds of investigations demonstrate that the impact of the environment has to be considered in understanding the workings of the brain. Indeed, what we have learned is that there is remarkable plasticity in the human brain, so that it changes according to its use. As the German neurobiologist Gerald Huether observes, we have "a brain which to some degree first programs itself by the way in which it is used. So we must decide how and for what we use it."[26]

As creatures of God whose human nature is constituted by our standing in relationship to God and to our fellow human beings, we must also insist on the integrity of a sense of self that acts with purpose and intentionality. While the soul and mind are concepts that capture important aspects of our life and experience without denoting entities in themselves, the concept of self is different in that it denotes a body-self; it refers to our nature as embodied persons. Our self-knowledge is inextricable from our bodily identity, and as embodied selves, we are agents that act in the world and relate to God and other human beings. This means that "freedom of the will" is a meaningful concept for us as moral decision makers, not because we are disembodied souls unhindered by the constraints of the world, but precisely because we live in the midst of limitations and constraints and know the difference between coerced and uncoerced behavior. Freedom is an existential, experienced reality, reflecting a meaningful degree of autonomy for human beings as moral agents. This is not to deny that every choice we make restricts the options available to us, and that our embeddedness in the environment is a constraining factor, limiting our freedom by circumstances that coerce and restrain. Indeed, we are not as free as we might think we are, often being moved by subconscious or unconscious factors as well as unrecognized elements in the immediate and larger environment. Our rational nature, which we understand as our capacity for meaningful, purposive action, is not quite the captain of our fate that we assume it to be.

The fact remains, however, that we do act with intention and purpose and are appropriately regarded as accountable for the choices we make. It is not a matter of whether we are free in any absolute sense, but that we are sufficiently free to make moral responsibility a defining feature of what it means to be human; moral experience cannot be removed by "explaining" it in terms of a causal chain of neurobiological reactions. The moral life with its sense of obligation and responsibility is an essential part of the Christian's self-consciousness as a child of God. The question finally posed by scientific materialism is not whether an entity we call the soul or the mind exists, but whether our subjective experience involves what we think it does—experiencing the realities of the spiritual life, such as depending upon the grace of God, making meaningful choices that shape our lives according to goals and ideals, and relating to others in moral commitments that bring obligations and responsibilities. All of these rich facets of human experience are made possible by the incredibly complex organization of the human brain and neural system, responding to the manifold signals offered by the natural and cultural environment.

## Searching for the Biological Basis of Religion

The dramatic advances in neurobiology have led to a number of attempts to define and comprehend religion on the basis of what goes on in the brain. There can be an aura of momentous discovery and even revelation in these attempts. The fact that it is a "scientific" approach to religion confers an immediate status to these efforts; it carries significant promise of being a final word on the subject. The force of this point is enhanced by the fact that religious belief is a universal phenomenon in the story of humankind as well as a subject of considerable contention. It is understandable that researchers in the biosciences have found religion to be an inviting subject.

The notion that neurobiology can bestow a definitive word on religion is more than obvious in the title of Pascal Boyer's book *Religion Explained*. Boyer, a cognitive anthropologist, bases his conclusions about religion on evolutionary biology and neuroscience. He concludes, "There is no religious instinct, no *specific* inclination in the mind, no particular disposition for [religious] concepts, no special religion center in the brain."[27] He identifies brain modules that have developed over the course of human evolution as problem solvers for different kinds of challenges arising in the environment. These modules have been formed from prehistoric times, creating mental organization or "inference systems" in the brain that lead people to behave in certain ways. In the case of religious ideas, they have emerged from the brain's response to human vulnerability. Gods and spirits are not inventions "out of the blue" but the product of inferences concerning distant threats to our well-being. It is significant that what Boyer has learned about the brain's inferential systems as the source of religious ideas also provides him with an interpretation of religion: it becomes a "mere consequence or side effect" of the way the brain functions.[28]

David J. Linden, professor of neuroscience at the Johns Hopkins University School of Medicine, also proceeds from the brain as a basis for his conclusions on religion; he agrees with Boyer that there is no point in looking for a particular region of the brain or a neurotransmitter or gene "that somehow confers religion":

> Rather let's ask: are there some aspects of brain function that, *on the average*, make it easy for humans to acquire and transmit religious thought? I will try to convince you that our brains have become particularly adaptive to creating coherent, gap-free stories and that this propensity for narrative creation is part of what predisposes humans to religious thought.[29]

While both of these scholars focus on the brain as the source of the religious impulse, the meaning or interpretation of what the brain is telling us is quite different in each case. This fact points to the Achilles' heel in this kind of approach. While scientific work always involves interpretation, deriving a religious "message" from the brain poses a most formidable challenge. Given the disparity among conclusions on this subject, one is inclined to say that any interpretation is likely to tell us more about the scientist than what one gleans from the brain. Linden's interpretation, including his observation that "our brains have evolved to make us believers," might indicate an interpretation that is friendlier to religious belief than Boyer's, but in any event, everything lies in the interpretation one makes of an inherently obscure piece of information.

This fact is further illustrated in the recent phenomenon called "neurotheology." As in the preceding two cases, neurotheology places the biological source of human spirituality in the brain, but it makes a particular point of repudiating those who would explain away the meaning and integrity of spiritual experience by reducing it to the physicochemical reactions that occur there. To do so would betray an imperialist attitude on the part of science that fails to recognize its own limitations:

> The organizing principle of science declares that everything that is real can be measured, and scientific methods are the only measurements that count. So whatever can't be measured, weighed, counted, scanned, or otherwise analytically understood by scientific methods cannot, with any confidence, be called real. Science alone can recognize reality.[30]

Advocates of neurotheology not only reject this materialist belief, but seek to "advance the exploration of the intersection of science and religion in a way that allows each perspective to enhance, rather than diminish, the other."[31] Through their research, they hope to shed new light on the origins of spirituality as well as bring increased scientific insights into the "mysterious workings" of the human brain. Scientists Andrew Newberg and Eugene D'Aquili use the latest imaging technology to study the brain during mystical contemplation, monitoring blood flow and measuring neural activity in different areas of the brain during these heightened moments of meditation. The assumption is that these intense experiences are on the far end of a continuum that includes the more "ordinary" spiritual experiences of people of faith, associated, for example, with prayer, hymn singing, and the reading of Scripture.

While the believer can appreciate the positive perspective that neurotheology brings to the subject, the temptation, once again, is to think that the brain sciences can provide a final word on not only the origins but the meaning of spiritual experiences. The authors of *Why God Won't Go Away* speak of a "religious urge" that is universal and the "driving spiritual force" behind all religions, believing that empirical means of investigating that urge may shed new light on the common ingredients of all religion, whether it be myth, ritual, or mystical experience. They believe that their research may establish a "megatheology" that is based on the universal characteristics of all religion, promising new insight into the beliefs of particular religions. For example, exploring the Christian dogma of the Holy Trinity from a biological perspective may not solve the ontological issue involved, but it may provide important information that could shed some light on the meaning of the dogma. A similar case could apply to myths, which often resolve seemingly irreconcilable opposites. Understanding how the brain helps us resolve such problems may enhance theology in bringing new insight and understanding to the promises of religion.[32]

Despite the good intentions, I'm afraid one has to respond to neurotheology with considerable skepticism. It promises more than it can deliver with its attempt to bring biological answers to questions of theology. It raises in a different form the difficulty I've noted earlier: the logical problem in moving from the realm of neurobiology to the realm of the mental life and questions of faith. While neurotheologians are not guilty of the kind of imperialism they identify with scientism, they do reflect the common assumption that the biosciences are where one finds definitive answers to most everything concerning humanity, including the religious life. A more promising approach to understanding the phenomenon of religion is to address the macro realm of human interaction, involving the life of personal and communal relationships in all of their psychological and social dimensions. This moves us from the natural sciences to the social sciences and humanities, to philosophy and theology, where the subject matter and methodologies are far more promising to a fruitful study of the religious life.

Obviously, the brain is involved in religious experience, but to say that the brain is the *source and cause* of religious experience is to oversimplify. It implies that religious experience is *produced* by the brain, as though we were addressing religious life in a vacuum. On the contrary, religious life occurs within a cultural environment, and we can say that our brains and neural systems enable us to respond to signals in the environment that elicit a religious experience. This means that there is no "generic religion" out there, divorced from history. For Christians, it is the biblical witness proclaimed by the church that shapes the nature of their religious experience, while the Hindu experience is quite different in its response to the sacred writings of the *Bhagavad Gita*. The religious "urge" previously noted does not take a generic form but is identified with the concepts generated by one's religious tradition. We might say that the *capacity* for a religious response is embedded in our human nature, but its expression always involves interpretation that is shaped by the religious tradition we inherit or make our own. Religious experience is a two-way street.

A second observation, not always acknowledged by those who engage in neurotheology, is that any claim that human religiosity is wired into our makeup does not constitute a proof for the existence of God or a guarantee of the validity of religious belief. Whatever role the brain might play in generating transcendental experience, the experience itself is always subject to interpretation; what goes on in the brain does not verify or prove the metaphysical reality of the referent to which the experience relates. One's conclusion on this matter will reveal the convictions that one brings to it, with some finding support for their faith in the knowledge that they are neurologically inclined toward faith, while others read this fact as evidence that religious faith is a deception encouraged by our neurological makeup.[33] In any event, issues of faith and unbelief are addressed with far more cogency at the level of human consciousness and personal relationships than at the cellular level.

## Concluding Thoughts

The reductionist principle that underlies scientific materialism has been debated among scientists themselves in recent years.[34] A major argument is that laws governing biological activities at the molecular level cannot adequately explain more complex levels of organization. If biological evolution is a "story in progress," or an ongoing process characterized by increasing levels of complexity, it can be logically understood in terms of the higher levels of organization that are attained rather than by lower levels of organization. This position is argued by philosopher Holmes Rolston III: "Nature and history have been creative, making more out of less. The essential characteristic of narrative is that events have to be understood in the light of the complexities to which they lead, not just in the light of the origins from which they flow. The event structures toward which they climb, their endings, are as significant as the matter-energy out of which they arise, their beginnings."[35] This approach not only gives priority, quite appropriately, to what we know and experience in the macro world, but also recognizes the open-ended character of human nature—an important dimension of the Christian understanding. Christian thinking follows a futurist direction: to ask who we are is to ask who we will become, ultimately turning us to a destiny that transcends death itself.

The scientist-theologian Ian Barbour makes some helpful observations that are directly applicable to our subject here. He notes the appeal of new paradigms that emerge on the scientific frontier, capturing the imaginations of scientists and philosophers of science, who then apply the new model to a broader understanding of our world and the place of human beings within it. This was the case in the eighteenth century, when many believed that Newtonian physics could account for all phenomena, giving us a cosmological key that would enable us to predict all future happenings. Twentieth-century quantum physics provided a new model for understanding the micro world that challenged these conclusions. Now, says Barbour, molecular biology has emerged as a tremendously fruitful research program, tempting thinkers to believe it can reveal and explain every facet of human behavior. However, new ideas in the biosciences are already challenging this reductionist thinking. I would conclude, together with Barbour, that the concept of *holism* proves to be far more fruitful than its opposite, reductionism, in understanding human nature. According to the holistic view, we do not understand the whole by analyzing its parts, but the whole is more than the sum of its parts and actually affects the behavior of its parts.[36] Holism recognizes the emergence of that which is new in the process of evolution, bringing new directions and new capacities that in turn affect the organism and shape its future.

My conclusion is that any claim that all of life's events, including human self-awareness, behavior, and cultural achievements, can ultimately be explained by an argument of causality based on molecular activity simply lacks credibility. Recent decades have seen increasing resistance to this supposedly scientific paradigm that results in neurobiological determinism. Scientists themselves are readier today to recognize the self-direction and creative interaction with the environment that characterize the more complex organization seen in human beings and the culture in which they move. It is a dialectical relationship between organism and environment, person and society. As humans, we bring our genetic identity to society, but at the same time, that identity is not formed in isolation but as a consequence of social life. This dialectical relation means that both the monist understanding, whether from "below" or from "above," and the dualist understanding are inadequate and misleading. While this "two-way street" applies to all organisms, it takes on a unique character with human beings. With increasing cognitive ability comes increasing flexibility and creativity in responding to one's needs and to the environment. At the level of human activity, marked by language and self-transcendence, self-direction and purposive behavior become distinguishing characteristics that are indispensable to our understanding of human nature.[37]

An aspect of this subject worth noting is the encouragement that a dualistic position has given to biological determinism. A body devoid of spiritual interest becomes a machine operating according to causal laws. This was Descartes's conclusion in his separation of the soul from the body, and this metaphor of the machine continues to dominate science in its view of organic life. It understands the human being in terms of its parts, which is the way we understand a machine. If we are willing to see human life as more than "molecules in motion," we can adopt either a dualism of matter and spirit or, as I am arguing, a psychosomatic, holistic view that recognizes the spirit-character of our being as a body-self in relationship. This latter view is true to our experience and provides an authentic expression of both our biological and our spiritual nature. Our understanding of human nature in terms of relatedness also expresses our engagement with the world more adequately, identifying us with the world in our mortality and turning us to God as the source of a transcendent hope by which we can live.

My consideration of the apparent conflict between science and religion in this chapter has focused primarily on the "mind/body problem," raising the question as to how the physical operations of the brain and neural system are related to our subjective experience. We have seen how this question can be seductive, leading us from the realm of scientific, inductive reasoning to the realm of ideology and the attempt to explain and define human consciousness exclusively in terms of physiological processes. The problem is that we cannot translate psychology into biology without losing what we perceive to be uniquely important dimensions of human nature and our sense of identity. Such a mistake not only violates logic but also carries destructive implications for our understanding of human nature. The description of physiological processes cannot begin to do justice to what we would call the depth dimension of human life—our religious and moral experience and all that it brings to life lived in relationship. To limit ourselves to the language of biology and genetics is to severely flatten the language necessary to an adequate portrayal of what it means to be human.

Though any predictions concerning a subject of this kind are precarious, one wonders whether we will ever resolve the mind/body issue in any definitive way. I would suggest that the best we can say is that they are two aspects of the same reality that require two different kinds of language. Our self-awareness and subjective consciousness are immediate, intimate, and personal, requiring the language that expresses these dimensions of the interior life. Scientific investigation of the brain involves the world of empirical data, the exterior world that is understood as object rather than subject, requiring a quite different language. The validity in Wilson's concern to bring sociology and biology together is not to be found by reducing the one to the other, but by affirming our social and biological nature as a holistic unity that rules out both reductionist and dualist fallacies.

CHAPTER 3

# Human Nature and the Gene

Genetics is a relatively new arrival among the disciplines that make up the natural sciences. The name was first suggested by William Bateson in 1906, and now a century later, it has moved from humble beginnings to a dominant, cutting-edge role in both science and the larger life of society. We can define genetics as the biological science that deals with heredity: the nature and function of the biological material that transmits inherited characteristics. This definition, however, does not begin to convey the full range of genetics today; it has moved well beyond its classical boundaries of heredity and cytology (the study of cellular life), becoming a core element of biology itself. While genetics is a basic science, its application has extended to agriculture in connection with the breeding of plants and animals, to industry in the many expressions of biotechnology, and to the practice of medicine in efforts to improve human health. Paleontology, archaeology, and forensics are but a few of the disciplines in which genetics plays a decisive role. Few if any scientific and technological enterprises garner as much public attention today as do genetics and the biotechnologies it has spawned. In the coming decades, we face the prospect of momentous changes to our bodies and to our mental and emotional life that will challenge our sense of self-identity and our understanding of human nature. Genetics will play a prominent role in these developments, so this science deserves special attention in any consideration of human nature and identity.

For those who are not well versed in genetics—and I am presuming that the reader is among them—it is helpful first to get some sense of the historical background to the emergence of genetics as we know it today, as well as some knowledge about the genetic makeup of the human body. The story of genetics is fascinating, involving many scientists over the past century and a half, each making a particular contribution that has supplied another piece in figuring out the puzzle. That puzzle—the genetic makeup of human beings and its implications for medicine—is still in the process of being solved; current developments are so swift that anyone who writes on the subject risks being out of date even while writing. Here, quite briefly, are some features of the historical background.

## From Mendel to Watson and Crick

The first significant figure in the story of genetics is the Austrian monk Gregor Mendel (1822–1884). This humble brother was a passionate gardener with an insatiable curiosity about the different varieties of pea plants in his garden. He embarked on a massive experiment in hybridizing pea plants, meticulously recording characteristics of plants, flowers, pods, and seeds from generation to generation. He concluded (contrary to the conclusions of Charles Darwin at the time) that hereditary characteristics do not "mix," but pop up as discrete features in each succeeding generation of plants. Mendel concluded that the structure of each plant contains hereditary elements (what he called "germinal units"), discrete entities that came to be called genes. It appeared that, just as the world of physics had its atoms, the world of biology now had its genes. In 1865 Mendel published a description of his work in a relatively obscure journal, and it went unnoticed. It was not until 1900 that the significance of his work was recognized, and in the years that followed, scientists concluded that he had indeed provided an accurate description of the building blocks of our hereditary makeup. As to their actual content and function, however, those blocks remained a mystery.

Further experimentation established the fact that genes are not unchangeable. The biologist Hermann Muller earned a Nobel Prize by bombarding fruit flies with X-rays, discovering in the process that genes are mutable—they can be artificially changed. This discovery sparked intense interest in the nature of the gene; it was clearly seen to be a source of action, but what action and how? In the 1940s, George Beadle and Edward Tatum concluded that genes control biochemical reactions through enzymes, a form of protein that functions like a catalyst. Did this mean that genes themselves are proteins? Already in the late nineteenth century, it was determined that chromosomes, which are linear strands within the nucleus of the cell that carry the hereditary genes, contain an acid called deoxyribonucleic acid, or DNA (a nucleic acid containing the sugar deoxyribose). DNA had been isolated by a Swiss doctor named Friedrich Miescher in 1869, but its role was not clear. In 1892 Miescher himself opined in a letter to his uncle that DNA might constitute the "language" by which heredity is conveyed in the human organism. It was a remarkable calculation that some fifty years later was proven to be correct. In 1943 researchers at the Rockefeller Institute determined that DNA is linked to the passing on of genetic information to each generation of an organism. But how does this occur?

A huge step toward answering this question came in 1953. At the Cavendish Laboratory of the University of Cambridge, an American biologist, James Watson, collaborated with an English physicist turned biologist, Francis Crick, in discovering the structure of DNA, which enabled them to discern how DNA is replicated. That event has been described as the greatest scientific discovery of the century, if not the millennium. The two scientists described the DNA model in a one-page paper, published in the journal *Nature*; it opened up an incredibly rich pathway to many more biological and biomedical breakthroughs.

## Structure and Function of DNA

DNA is a molecule that looks like a ladder or spiral staircase with two twists in it—what Watson and Crick called a "double helix." It is tightly coiled at several levels in the nucleus of the cell. The two sides of the ladder are composed of sugar and phosphate components that carry nucleotides, or chemical compounds. The nucleotides constitute the rungs of the ladder, protruding inward, and are arranged in pairs called bases; they constitute the most important part of DNA. The bases number some three billion, but just a small percentage seems to be involved in gene activity. Whereas genes had been regarded as discrete units of hereditary material, Watson and Crick's observations showed that they are minute sections of DNA. Just how many genes there are in the human genome was debated, and until quite recently most geneticists believed, mistakenly, that the number was in the neighborhood of 100,000. The information or code that they contain spells out the recipes for proteins, which are essential to the growth and restoration of bodily tissue.

It was not until the 1960s that the DNA code was cracked, enabling us to understand how DNA passes on the information that enables organisms to function. The process involves replication, in which the base pairs in a DNA molecule, formed from the nucleotides identified as adenine (A), cytosine (C), guanine (G), and thymine (T), project from the sides of the ladder to connect with each other. The nucleotide A is always paired with T, and C with G, but in a different order from one molecule to the next. Their interconnection results in the replication of new DNA cells that are faithful copies of the original. The ordering of the bases, which are arranged in groups of three (for example, ATG GTA GAC TGC . . .), results in the production of each of the twenty amino acids. Cracking the genetic code involved determining which order or sequence of the bases in the DNA (called a "codon") resulted in the forming of each of the amino acids, which in turn assemble into a wide variety of proteins that carry out the work of the organism.

These chemical processes at the molecular level (described here in much abbreviated fashion) provide the basis for all the complex actions of a living being. At the risk of oversimplifying, we might say that genes tell cells how to behave, what proteins to make, and when to start and stop growing. Every metaphor is inadequate, but Ian Barbour suggests the following language:

> In the DNA, then, an "alphabet" of just four "letters" (A, C, G, and T bases), grouped in three-letter "words" (each specifying one of the amino acids), is arranged in "sentences" (specifying

particular proteins). Thousands of sentences of varying length and word order can be made from the twenty basic words, so there are thousands of possible proteins. Long paired strands, made of exactly the same four bases in various sequences, constitute the genes of all organisms, from microbes to human beings. In all known organisms, the same code is used to translate from DNA to protein, which seems to indicate a common origin for all living things.[1]

The important result of this molecular activity is the action it generates, with genes forming and directing the proteins that enable life processes to take place, whether these be breathing, body movement, thinking, or digestion. In generating this activity, genes themselves must be activated, or "switched on," by enzymes (proteins that allow specific chemical actions to occur more easily). The switched-on gene forms not only other proteins but also the complementary strand mRNA, which conveys the DNA in the formation of new proteins. In this way, the order and stability of organic life are transmitted within the constant division and adaptation of cells. While there is remarkable stability and constancy in this complicated process, there is occasional dissonance, which occurs when a gene undergoes a mutation, or change, where one letter in the three-letter code receives a substitute letter that may alter the production of proteins. Mutations are permanent changes in the DNA that can be harmful and cause a defect or a genetic disease. They may also be beneficial, however, if they create a new metabolic activity.

## Continuing Questions about the Gene

The preceding discussion about DNA has been purely descriptive, with no reference to issues of understanding and interpretation that are present in the scientific community. In fact, some scientists question whether the public discussion carried on in the media concerning the gene is contributing to considerable misunderstanding. Given the extensive publicity surrounding the Human Genome Project (discussed in the next section), which has prompted a steady stream of articles in the press, these scientists question whether all the excitement may be due to false assumptions concerning the gene. Not only our understanding of what is meant by the gene, but also our expectations concerning the potential benefits of genetic research, is at the center of this discussion.

Among scientists expressing these concerns has been Evelyn Fox Keller, professor of history and philosophy of science at Massachusetts Institute of Technology. Keller notes, as we have seen, that Mendelian genetics encouraged the notion of the gene as a discrete element or particle that functions autonomously. With the discovery of the structure of DNA and the nature of genetic material, that understanding was modified; as we noted, the gene was recognized as a minute segment of DNA. Another fact that was not easy for biologists to recognize was the inherently dynamic, volatile nature of DNA; the hereditary stability demonstrated in organisms belied this underlying frenzy of activity at the microscopic level.[2] Beyond this discovery, Keller argues, the inherent complexity of genetic material actually challenges the language we use in describing genes and what they do. As an example, she cites a 1957 comment from Francis Crick: "DNA makes RNA, RNA makes protein, and proteins make us."[3] This succinct description gives the impression that human beings are the sum of a series of pretty straightforward biochemical processes. The reality, however, is much more complex.

What we are learning, notes Keller, is that genes have multiple functions. In addition to the "structural" genes that are responsible for the proteins needed by the body (coding genes), there are also "regulator" genes whose function is to control the process. These noncoding genes turn the coding genes on and off and tweak them to make one version of a protein rather than another. It appears that only 5 percent of the DNA molded by evolution actually carries instructions for making proteins. While the other 95 percent of the DNA is involved in regulating gene activity, there is still much to learn about the full scope of what it does. Until recently, this vast majority of genetic material was summarily called "junk DNA" because it was assumed to be hereditary material that no longer had a function, but this view has changed. A further result of these discoveries is that scientists have discarded the belief that each gene produces its own particular protein. Now it appears that a hundred or more proteins can be associated with a given gene. It has also become clear that one protein may be carrying out many functions. In short, argues Keller, the very concept of the gene may be an anachronism; it once served a useful purpose, but now that usefulness may be outgrown.

Nonetheless, the word *gene* will continue to be used because it is so deeply embedded in biology as well as popular discourse, and as a kind of shorthand, it remains a helpful concept. The real challenge for society is to gain a more accurate grasp of the gene's complexity in order to avoid misunderstandings and questionable implications. These misunderstandings are particularly important in regard to claims concerning the impact of particular genes on human behavior. While scientists have succeeded in isolating genes connected to certain diseases, the picture is quite different when it comes to matching genes with the much more complex character of personality and behavior. The public seems to have adopted a common assumption that a particular gene can be found to account for every conceivable human characteristic, whether qualities of one's physical constitution or personality traits. Much popular discussion reflects the belief that there is a gene "for" this and "for" that, accounting for the totality of our physical and personal makeup. This idea is promulgated by the media, which avidly report the latest findings of "genetic researchers" that suggest an influential connection between one's genes and any number of personal attitudes, ranging from one's stance on social issues to one's commitment to marital fidelity to one's propensity toward risk-taking and violent behavior.

These deductions are appealing to many people because they provide clear reasons for particular behaviors and satisfy our desire to find answers to issues that otherwise appear formidably complex. This kind of thinking also reflects the impact of anything emanating from the scientific establishment, which carries considerable weight in our society. Scientists themselves, however, are far from agreement on these kinds of conclusions that would indicate a straight line from genes to behavior. Such thinking is "fanciful," according to biologist Ruth Hubbard, reflecting false conclusions about the power and control exercised by our genes. In fact, genes play "a crucial role, but a limited one. Many things that have nothing to do with genes affect the ways we develop and function day by day."[4] Hubbard argues that it is more realistic to think of genes as *participating* in various bodily reactions rather than *controlling* them. The consensus today is that DNA is both inherited and environmentally responsive, which raises the larger question of the interaction between organisms and their environment. Before we turn to that subject, it will be helpful to briefly describe what we have learned from that most unusual scientific accomplishment of our time, the Human Genome Project.

## The Human Genome Project

The human genome refers to the full complement of genes in the human organism, and the Human Genome Project (HGP) sent a clear signal that the genomic era was well under way. Where genetics has been the study of inherited traits, focusing on one gene or at most several genes at a time, genomics brings a broader picture of what all the genes in a cell are doing and how their activities are related. The science of genomics involves the decoding of the genomes of organisms stretching from single-celled bacteria to the human being, giving scientists a far more precise understanding of basic cell operations and the mechanics of natural selection.

As the knowledge of genomics has deepened and grown, it has impelled an obvious question: Can our greater understanding of the human genome enable medicine to effectively address the ravages of genetic disease? We know of more than four thousand genetic diseases, each involving one or more malfunctioning genes. Those genes could presumably be located and dealt with therapeutically by mapping and sequencing the DNA, but that task appeared insuperable because of the huge number of nucleotides or bases that constitute DNA—some three billion. It is estimated that if the nucleotides were typed in order, using their initial letters (A, C, G, and T), the sequence of bases would fill the equivalent of 134 complete sets of the *Encyclopaedia Britannica*. However, as noted in the previous section, just a small percentage of all DNA is active in the production of proteins, so the task involves locating the genes that are active and involved in affecting the health of the organism. Given the formidable difficulty up to the 1980s in attempting to sort out just a few hundred genes, that task appeared to be impossible. In addition, there were still other unknowns in our genetic knowledge: we were not clear on what the genome might contain, and much remained to be learned concerning the nature of genes themselves.

At this point, technology came to the rescue. With the invention of an automated DNA sequencer in 1986, the possibility of sequencing the whole human genome became conceivable. Four years later, the HGP was under way. Leroy Hood, a biologist at the California Institute of Technology, developed a method with his sequencer in which a different color of fluorescent dye was used to identify each of the four DNA bases, and a laser beam caused the dyes to glow. That glow was then fed as digital information directly into a computer. By 1999, a fully automated instrument was able to sequence up to 150 million base pairs annually, and now it is actually possible to sequence a whole human genome in two months, a time span that will undoubtedly continue to shrink. The other task, called mapping the genome, provided clues to where specific pieces of DNA belong by relating them to other markers on the chromosome. This helped to locate disease-causing genes that would be uncovered by sequencing, completing the overall task. At the outset, the HGP was planned to last fifteen years, but the development of further techniques and competition from the private sector led to a substantial completion of the work within ten years. A ceremony held in the White House in June 2000 recognized the supreme achievement of this three-billion-dollar, international project. On the occasion, the director of the project, Francis S. Collins, said, "It's a happy day for the world. It is humbling for me, and awe-inspiring, to realize that we have caught the first glimpse of our own instruction book, previously known only to God."[5]

What have we learned from the HGP? There were some surprising results on several fronts. Where the number of protein-coding genes in the human organism had been estimated at close to 100,000 or more, it became clear that the actual number is far less—estimates range from 22,000 to 30,000. Since this number brings humans into the range of worms, flies, and even plants, it's obvious that the meaning of genes derives from much more than a simple count of their number. It has become clear that the way the information in genes is utilized in an organism forms a critical part of the organism's complexity. Genes in lower creatures just don't perform the tasks they carry out in the human organism. Another discovery is that at the level of our DNA, humans are remarkably identical. Not only do we clearly belong to one family, but the genetic diversity within that family runs appreciably less than the diversity found in most other species, where it can be anywhere from ten to fifty times greater than among humans.[6] The many efforts throughout history to make distinctions between societies so that some can claim superiority over others receive precious little help from genetics. The evidence powerfully supports the common origin and identity of all human beings.

This means that the HGP further corroborates what we have learned from other sources concerning human origins. Population geneticists are agreed that our species has descended from ancestors who lived about 150,000 to 200,000 years ago. This conclusion coincides with the fossil record, which places the likely location of those ancestors in the area of East Africa. In addition, what we've learned from the HGP is that the match between the coding regions of DNA (leading to protein production) in humans and other mammals runs at a higher percentage than it does between their noncoding regions. In the case of mice, the similarity runs at 99 percent in coding regions and 40 percent in noncoding regions; for chickens, the figures are 75 percent and 4 percent. What does this mean? It gives still further credence to the notion of a common ancestry for all of God's creatures, as well as support for Darwin's notion of "a tree of life" that relates all living species. The evidence from genetics, the fossil record, and comparative anatomy all leads us to the same conclusion concerning human origins.[7]

As far as combating genetic diseases is concerned, the knowledge gained from the HGP has led researchers to project that eventually it will be common for people with a family history of genetic disease to have their own genome sequenced and mapped, providing information that will enable them to receive more effective medical treatment. Thus, individualized genetic therapy will become a much more powerful instrument in combating disease. A significant contributor to this development has been the tremendous progress in DNA-scanning technology, which has opened the door to a flood of new information on genetic links to a large variety of diseases. Scientists are now able to scan the entire complement of DNA in thousands of people, comparing the results from healthy subjects with those from people afflicted with genetic diseases. This is enabling them to pursue much more efficiently any deviations in the base pairs that can signal a genetic disease.

One can appreciate the excitement generated by these remarkable advances in our knowledge of the human genome. It represents an immense rising tide in our understanding of the biology of many diseases, which will in turn have a significant impact on the development of new therapies. Unfortunately, the promise of these developments is not likely to be fulfilled for many years, since most of the scientific work is still at the laboratory stage and years away from being clinically available. This situation has created an ethical issue related to genetic screening and testing: the ability of science to diagnose a disease is much more advanced than its ability to cure it, so testing in many cases serves no legitimate purpose. It gives patients knowledge of their disease with no real prospect of a cure. This problem has become more serious with the proliferation of genetic tests; at the cost of hundreds of dollars, one can now order tests online or through the mail, but the knowledge one gains is of little worth without the assistance of a doctor or genetic counselor to provide needed perspective. Unfortunately, the lure of big profits for biotech companies is overwhelming a rational approach and better judgment on the use of these instruments.

## Interaction of Organism and Environment

The achievement of the HGP and the promise it holds for improving the human condition are reasons enough for people to be greatly impressed with what genetics can accomplish. But the impact of the gene goes well beyond the realm of science, raising serious philosophical and theological questions about human nature. Many of these questions relate to the issue of biological reductionism discussed in the previous chapter, but with a focus on our genetic inheritance and the role it plays in shaping who we are. The question it raises is one that is often heard: Are we the product of our genes? Achieving the complete sequencing of the human genome had been anticipated by some scientists as the final answer to that question; in the words of the prominent molecular biologist Walter

Gilbert, "We will know what it is to be human."[8] This belief reflects the assumption that we are the "sum of our genes," organisms literally produced according to the instructions encoded in our genes when we were born.

Every discussion of DNA runs the risk of conveying this idea, because the subject is typically treated apart from any reference to a surrounding context. Attention understandably focuses on the inner workings of the genetic material in an effort to comprehend its nature. My own description here of DNA, amino acids, and proteins could easily give the impression that I have given the whole picture of what human life is really about. As noted in the earlier section on continuing questions, however, the notion that gene activity is a self-enclosed, linear process is a misconception. But the problem really goes deeper than this, revealing both an issue of scientific understanding and a critical philosophical issue. Biologists widely assume that the development of an individual is the unfolding of a predetermined genetic program. Wherever variations occur, they are accounted for by gene mutations, an approach that reinforces the belief that any variation of *phenotype* in respect to an individual's appearance and behavior must be due to one's *genotype*, or one's genetic makeup. One can see how this understanding encourages a genetic determinism in which the organism is a self-contained unit, fully explainable in terms of its genes. This kind of thinking finds eloquent expression in the works of Richard Dawkins, author of *The Selfish Gene* and soul brother, we might say, of Edward O. Wilson. He shares with Wilson the belief that molecular biology and genetics provide the definitive word in understanding who we are as human beings.

Many scientists have challenged this genetic reductionism, but their voices generally do not get as much media attention. A particularly forceful critic has been the evolutionary biologist Richard Lewontin, Alexander Agassiz Research Professor at the Museum of Comparative Zoology, Harvard University. He takes issue with the notion that who we become can be explained as a development of what is already present in our genes:

> The trouble with the general scheme of explanation contained in the metaphor of development is that it is bad biology. If we

had the complete DNA sequence of an organism and unlimited computational power, we could not compute the organism, because the organism does not compute itself from its genes. Any computer that did as poor a job of computation as an organism does from its genetic "program" would be immediately thrown into the trash and its manufacturer would be sued by the purchaser.[9]

In contrast to the gene-centered, developmental view, Lewontin points to the large body of evidence demonstrating that the ontogeny (origin and development) of the organism is "the consequence of a unique interaction between the genes it carries, the temporal sequence of external environments through which it passes during its life, and random events of molecular interactions within individual cells."[10]

The conclusion to be drawn from these observations is that a gene- or DNA-centered view of human nature is not only inadequate but also seriously misleading in its failure to recognize the complicated interaction of organism and environment in human development. A common fallacy in the understanding of biological evolution is to treat the environment as an autonomous entity that is separate from the organism. The organism is then challenged to adapt if it is going to survive. This view overlooks the fact that organisms themselves are active in defining their environment. They "create, destroy, modify, and internally transform aspects of the external world by their own life activities," entering into the making of their environment.[11] Of course, the genetic constitutions of the lion and the horse differ, accounting for their differences, but genes tell us little about the variations that occur within each of these, or any other, species. The fact that organisms are active in causing their environments applies to all forms of life in the evolutionary chain. The conscious action of human beings in particular has had a profound effect on the environment, creating "a dialectical development of organism and milieu in response to each other."[12]

What we are addressing here has often been termed the "nature versus nurture" debate, but one can see how framing the issue in these terms fails to recognize the complexity of the subject. It assumes two distinct and opposite sources of influence when it is impossible to work with that assumption. It leads to ill-advised attempts to determine the proper ratio between nature and nurture in shaping the individual phenotype—60 percent nature and 40 percent nurture, for example, or perhaps just the opposite, depending on the authority to whom one is listening. To avoid this fallacy, we might need a stronger word than *interaction* between organism and environment, such as the *interpenetration* of nature and nurture, of organism and environment.[13] We see genetic determinism versus cultural determinism at the opposite extremes of this debate, but neither captures the dialectical relation between ourselves and our environment. We are not autonomous selves that simply react to the environment, both natural and social, but are interdependent selves actively engaged in forming our environment even as we are being formed by it.[14]

A notable challenge to the idea of genetic causality has recently been expressed in the concept of *epigenetics* (perhaps best translated as "beyond genetics"). This term points to gene-modifying factors in human development, but scientists disagree about the implications of the concept. I refer to it here because some see it as a promising new paradigm in biology that broadens our understanding of the human genome in a radically holistic fashion. In contrast to any notion of genetic determinism, epigenetics refers to highly complex regulatory networks in cells and organisms that interact both internally and with the external environment. Each organism's adaptation to the environment is a creative process, *already at the cellular level*, with some scholars going so far as to adopt the metaphor of "choice" to describe what is going on in the basic functioning of organisms. Here is another challenge, this time from cellular biologists, to the notion that organisms develop in a one-dimensional fashion according to instructions in the DNA. Where it has been assumed that genes exercise exclusive control of the phenotype, we are now looking elsewhere in the cell for the control and assembly of vast amounts of information coming from the organism, including our thoughts and feelings. This epigenetic paradigm provides a scientific framework that is able to accommodate notions of purpose and intentionality that are essential to our understanding of human nature.[15]

## A God Gene?

I've noted (in chapter 2) the attempt of neurotheologians to find a source for the religious life in the brain. Perhaps not surprisingly, the same attempt has been made through investigation of our DNA. The noted geneticist Dean Hamer has written a book provocatively entitled *The God Gene: How Faith Is Hardwired into Our Genes*, in which he would trace human spirituality to our genetic makeup.[16] Unfortunately, the title is not only provocative but also misleading; by page 8, we are told that "the term 'God gene' is, in fact, a gross oversimplification" and that "environmental influences are just as important as genetics." Not even scientists can avoid false advertising for the sake of selling their books! Rather than faith being "hardwired into our genes," Hamer concludes that the nature of the genetic origins of human spirituality can be seen as "soft" wiring, more as predisposition than finished reality.

The critical issue beyond the misrepresentation of his claim is whether Hamer makes a solid case in arguing for a "genetic component" to human spirituality. He acknowledges the considerable challenge not only in *defining* spirituality, given its diffuseness in terms of so many feelings, beliefs, and experiences associated with the term, but in *measuring* it, a capacity that is necessary to any scientific analysis. In measuring spirituality (which he would differentiate from religion), Hamer utilizes a questionnaire featuring a "self-transcendence" scale that would provide a yardstick for both *faith* as understood in Western religions, and the search for *enlightenment* in Eastern religions. The immediate question is whether a questionnaire can serve as a satisfactory scientific instrument in this context, offering a definitive result in measuring a subject like spirituality. The questionnaire's criterion in determining the nature of spirituality turns out to be a sense of "oneness with the world." This is an experience one associates with mysticism and contemplation, characteristic of religions of the East, but how meaningful is it for those reared in the historic religions of the West? Does oneness with the world begin to capture the religious experience of the Christian who identifies God's presence with the person of Jesus Christ, associating faith with discipleship and social justice rather than the life of a mystic?

This is not to rule out a sense of unity with the world as a theme that can be associated with Christian faith. It can be understood as a sense of completeness and fulfillment that captures a dimension of the emotional nature of religious experience, but it hardly gets at the distinctive nature of the Christian experience. That experience places one in the presence of divine grace and mercy as defined by, and embodied in, the life of Jesus. It carries the acknowledgment that one is a sinner in need of forgiveness and renewal, in contrast to the experience of unity with the world that assumes one's personal integrity and wholeness. The emotional power of the Christian experience lies in its recognition of one's brokenness and the need of forgiveness, and of the gift of wholeness bestowed by that forgiveness and renewal. At that point, the experience of one's wholeness and completeness is not "to become one with the universe and everybody and everything in it,"[17] but to enter into the presence of a merciful God who accepts the sinner and restores one to spiritual health. This point places in question the effort of Hamer to separate spirituality from religion, for one's religion in fact shapes and gives the peculiar content to one's spirituality. His assumption that spirituality has a genetic origin while religion belongs to environmental influences also lacks credibility; it betrays an effort to distinguish between nature and nurture in a way that is highly problematic. Given his understanding of spirituality, it is not surprising to learn that Hamer's experiments centered on the mystical exercises of Zen monks.[18]

Any consideration of Hamer's efforts to make a credible case for there being a "God gene" must make the same methodological point I made in chapter 2 in regard to neurotheology: attempts to explain or illuminate human spirituality or religious belief by conducting research at the molecular level fail to address the origins of either spirituality or religion. The fact that the human genome plays a role in all of life's experiences and the importance of the brain sciences for understanding some of the dynamics of the spiritual life go without saying, but their significance is limited to the biological realm. They become relevant when the body needs medical or psychiatric help to return to normal functioning. The origins, meaning, and importance of spirituality and religion can only be addressed at the level of human consciousness and in light of the personal and community relationships into which people enter. Anthropologist Barbara King has it right when she stresses "the primacy of the social, the emotional, the imaginative, and the transformative in explaining the origins of the religious imagination."[19]

## Genes, Culture, and Faith in God

The reductionist argument is made not only at the individual level in relation to the brain and human consciousness, but also at the level of human culture, reducing all cultural expressions ultimately to genetics. The argument of Richard Dawkins concerning the "selfish gene," shaping human behavior in a self-preserving way in order to survive (the principle of natural selection), moves to the level of culture with his concept of the "meme" as a unit of cultural transmission. Just as genes replicate themselves, so memes, whether as ideas, clothes fashions, tunes, or whatever, replicate themselves in a process of propagation from brain to brain. The meme, according to Dawkins, is an analogue of the gene, competing for survival in a process of natural selection within society's "cultural soup." As with Wilson, Dawkins maintains a degree of open-endedness in order to avoid the charge that human behavior is genetically determined, but any view of the human being that is based on molecular biology implies a determinism of cause and effect. A biological framework controls society at both the individual and cultural levels.

The implications of this view are disturbing, particularly in the realm of ethics. Dawkins's view of the selfish gene leads him to reject altruism as a meaningful or important concept in human interaction; it can only be regarded as an evolutionary dead end. While *altruism* is a modern word (coined by Auguste Comte) and not a simple equivalent of the biblical concept of *agapē*, or sacrificial love, both express an ideal that is quite the opposite of selfishness. How have believers been persuaded to accept an ideal that genetically they are moved to reject? Defenders of the Dawkins paradigm argue that the altruism of religion is actually a deception, a pseudo-altruism motivated by selfish reasons. The values of culture, including cooperation and respect for one's neighbor, are actually biological strategies that parade as ethical values, designed to further what best serves our own selfish interests.

In contrast to this remarkably cynical view, it is far more convincing to maintain that human ethics is not the product of biological evolution or of nature, but of human culture as it has evolved in history. Life together in society and the quest for community require different rules than genetics can offer. The ideal of altruism asks more of us than we are often willing to give, but we recognize its power and validity; where taken seriously, it inculcates a spirit that makes community possible, humanizing people in response to the requirements of society. Culture requires order in contrast to chaos, which in turn requires cooperation, respect of one's neighbor, rules of morality, and the inculcation of moral responsibility. All of the historic religions lift up the ideal of compassion for the stranger, teaching a universal morality that transcends the morality of the tribe. While religion is often distorted by the weaknesses of human nature, the net result of its impact has been to enhance culture through its humanizing influence.[20]

Richard Dawkins poses an interesting case of a scientist who is willing to enter the public forum and engage vigorously in philosophical warfare. While Edward O. Wilson is an advocate of scientific materialism, Dawkins has become a veritable missionary on behalf of atheism. I believe his stance reflects the vacuum of meaning in his concept of the selfish gene. To find the point of human existence at the level of one's DNA is bound to be a sterile enterprise; the secret of life turns out to be no more than the drive to survive. We are here to compete with everyone or anything that becomes an adversary, but the human question remains: For what purpose are we to survive? To define the ultimate goal of human life in terms of selfishness is to drain that life of the meaning and purpose we naturally seek. It is little wonder that Dawkins feels the urge to remove the principal threat to his gene-controlled universe: faith in God that moves one beyond the self-centered life to concern for one's neighbor and the world that nourishes us.

In his book *The God Delusion*,[21] Dawkins launches a full-fledged attack on the notion of God, portraying religious belief as not only delusional but even pernicious, an evil that threatens the very future of humanity. The popularity of his book (making the *New York Times* best-seller list and putting the author on the cover of *Time* magazine) is hardly warranted, however, in light of the amateurish way in which he engages his subject. Much of his attack is directed against a "straw man" version of religion, focusing on simplistic expressions of fundamentalism and biblical literalism. He seems to be neither acquainted with nor interested in the rich theological heritage of the Christian tradition, making no effort to come to grips with its more sophisticated insights into the human condition. Equally disconcerting is his tendency to treat atheism at the level of theory but religion at the level of practice, holding up all the warts and blemishes of human weakness that are manifest in the life of religion as a means of denigrating religious belief. When it comes to the horrors perpetrated by secularized totalitarian regimes such as Stalinist Russia, he refuses to draw the same kind of inferences that would link crimes against humanity with a militant atheism.[22] It is fair to say that the book lacks the objectivity we might expect from a person schooled in the sciences.

Dawkins's attempt to discredit belief in God warrants a response. My purpose here has been to spell out a view of human nature in conversation with genetics, rather than to defend the existence of God as such. At the same time, my view of human nature assumes the reality of God, making any atheistic argument a legitimate concern. The most we can do here is to indicate the direction of an appropriate response within the context of religion's encounter with science, recognizing that any intellectual argument on behalf of God is severely limited in view of the nature of faith, which is much more than an intellectual decision. Here again, it should be noted that the conflict over God is not between the believer and science as such, but between the believer's convictions and what scientists like Dawkins believe they can infer from the results of scientific investigation.

One must acknowledge at the outset that an appropriate Christian response is not to claim—as do the advocates of Intelligent Design—that science itself requires the inference that an intelligent designer has been at work. Such a claim destroys the assumption that is critical to the viability of the sciences, namely, that scientific explanations must be limited to natural causes within the empirical world. Nor can the Christian make the claim that goes back to medieval if not ancient times, that the existence of God can be proven by logical, deductive reasoning that proceeds from the empirical world to the necessity of a divine Cause.

There is no logical proof that would compel one to acknowledge the reality of God; indeed, that reality can hardly be affirmed apart from the movement within a person's life that we call faith, embracing the whole person in a deeply rooted commitment.

Despite my skepticism about arriving at God through intellectual argument, there are, nonetheless, some important things that can be said about the intelligibility of believing in God. They are evidences that support the venture of faith, but given the nature of that venture, they do not prove the reality of God to the skeptic. Among scientists who are believers, the fact that we live in a cosmos rather than chaos, a universe of rational order and predictable patterns that supports the kind of life we know and experience as human beings, is enough to inspire a sense of wonder and awe. Scientist Kenneth R. Miller puts it well:

> As more than one scientist has said, the truly remarkable thing about the world is that it actually makes sense. The parts fit, the molecules interact, the darn thing works. To people of faith, what evolution says is that nature is complete. God fashioned a material world in which truly free, truly independent beings could evolve. He got it right the very first time.[23]

When one moves beyond scientific explanations to the broader realm of human meaning and purpose, the theistic conclusion, as scientist John Polkinghorne observes, "can claim serious consideration as an intellectually satisfying understanding of what would otherwise be unintelligible good fortune." This assertion "in no way seeks to be a rival to scientific explanation but rather seeks to complement that explanation by setting it within a wider and more profound context of understanding."[24] That "wider and more profound context" includes the spiritual realities of, first, a value-laden world that inspires a quest for justice and, second, in the face of our mortality, the presence of hope that stretches beyond the grave. Both of these deeply personal experiences are central to the human struggle against nihilism and find their most powerful source and inspiration in God. While not a proof, this kind of reasoning can support faith and prompt serious reflection for the unbeliever.

This larger context in considering human nature adds to the discomfort one has with biological and genetic reductionism. Neo-Darwinism today, in the interpretation of scientists like Edward O. Wilson and Richard Dawkins, turns what is valid in natural selection into a universal principle of explanation that would account for everything we know about humanity. The inadequacy of their argument is particularly apparent when we consider human consciousness. Our awareness of vulnerability to present and future danger is obviously important to survival—a feature of our "fitness" in negotiating the environment—but human consciousness takes us far beyond what is demanded in the everyday struggle for survival. Turning to John Polkinghorne once more, he notes that when one considers, for example, mathematics and the mysteries it has unlocked about the subatomic world, or the ethical demand and the experience of altruism, or the astonishing creativity of humans in composing masterworks of art, music, and poetry, one is overwhelmed with the achievement these things represent and the profound enrichment they bring to the cultural environment. That environment moves one well beyond the categories of struggle and survival identified with Darwinian thinking, which is simply too restrictive to account for the breadth and depth of the culture created by the human community.[25]

## Concluding Thoughts

In this chapter, we have moved from biological to cultural evolution and have noted the attempt of a sociobiologist like Richard Dawkins to account for cultural evolution on the basis of principles rooted in genetics. I have argued that whether focusing on the individual and the nature of our humanity or on the culture formed by people in community, this approach cannot do justice to the issue of human nature. We are certainly shaped by our genes, but the question remains in what way. Genes establish the shape of one's nose and the color of one's hair, but when it comes to behavior, I believe scientist Stephen Jay Gould offers a helpful perspective. He places genetic influence in the context of "ranges" that would limit our behavior rather than "blueprints" that govern specific behaviors. He sees sociobiologists as setting a narrow enough range to lead them "to program a specific behavior as the predictable result of possessing certain genes."[26] Gould, in contrast, would place genetic influence at the "deeper level" of structures or rules that give rise to human behavior, rather than at the level of "products" of those structures, such as specific conditions or behaviors—Joe's homosexuality or Martha's shyness, for example. At most, Gould's point would lead one to ascribe genetic *predispositions* to certain behavior rather than infer that genes *determine* that behavior. In other words, genes are not destiny; they provide the range or the tendency, but it is up to us to chart the course.

When it comes to human culture, what sociobiologists fail to recognize is the qualitative difference that it introduces to our concept of evolution. (To avoid this confusion, Gould prefers the language of "cultural change" rather than cultural evolution.) Cultural evolution is built on human intelligence and the power it gives us in manipulating and changing the world. Biological evolution continues, but at an incomparably slower pace than for cultural evolution. The ability of humans to pass on what they have learned from generation to generation quickens immeasurably the pace of change while maintaining continuity. That change is rapid as well as reversible, introducing the concept of progress at the cultural level when it comes to the technological advancement of society.

An observation by Theodosius Dobzhansky, a key figure in the emergence of neo-Darwinism, expresses the qualitative change between biological and cultural evolution in the language of biology and genetics:

> Human genes have accomplished what no other genes succeeded in doing. They formed the biological basis for a super-organic culture, which proved to be the most powerful method of adaptation to the environment ever developed by any species. . . . The development of culture shows regularities *sui generis*, not found in biological nature, just as biological phenomena are subject to biological laws which are different from, without being contrary to, the laws of inorganic nature.[27]

The fascinating truth about human nature is that we come into the world in an unfinished state, becoming who we are through a process of culturalization that involves human relationships and moral and spiritual development. This process cannot be adequately explained by remaining at the level of biology, important as that level is for fully understanding who we are. Unlike the lower animals, ruled and limited by instinctual behavior, human beings reflect a complex level of consciousness that opens them to the future and to transcendence, generating a uniquely human response to God, to themselves, to each other, and to the natural environment. Genetics is at the basis of it all, the necessary substratum, but also just the beginning of a much more interesting and complicated story that takes us well beyond the reach of genetic explanation.

Another way of making this point is to say that we as humans are involved in two stories, both of which contribute to who we are. The larger story is that of nature, encompassing the whole universe but centering for us in the world made possible by God's "Mother Earth," generating life that has led to the marvelous story of the human being. This latter story is much more limited, embedded in the story of nature and constituting but a minute temporal fraction of that vast story. However, this second story that has emerged from the first is radically new, defining humans as creatures with self-consciousness who enter into relationships that create community and give human beings a past, present, and future. We can understand the perennial tension between science and religion as the result of attempts to define who we are in light of these two stories. The story of nature can be interpreted in ways that reduce humans to natural categories, whether in terms of molecular activity or an animal past. The obvious alternative proposed by people of faith and many others is to recognize the second story as that which truly defines us, embracing our biological past, our present experience, and the future that our evolution has made possible.

PART TWO

# Christian Faith and Our Biotech Future

CHAPTER 4

# Human Nature and the Impact of Biotechnology

As we turn to the challenges that biotechnology poses to human nature and identity, it will be helpful first to summarize the conclusions I have reached in the three preceding chapters. These conclusions concerning human nature provide a basis or point of orientation from which I address those challenges. My intent as a Christian theologian has been to understand who we are as human beings in light of what we know concerning our biological origins. Thus, my discussion to this point has leaned heavily on what we have learned from the biosciences, particularly evolutionary biology and genetics, with the intent to integrate their insights into a Christian understanding of human nature. At the same time, I have challenged those scientists who have adopted a materialistic or naturalistic point of view, a philosophical position they want to identify with science. This kind of discriminating conversation between religion and science is what a responsible Christian theology is intent on doing: to recognize truth wherever it is found and to relate our faith and theology to it; to respond critically and authentically to what we are learning and experiencing in today's world.

## Theses Concerning Human Nature

In the spirit of that conversation, I list here in summary fashion the conclusions I have reached concerning our understanding of human nature:

1. Christian anthropology must not reject or ignore the findings of the biosciences concerning human origins and the evolution of our species. Charles Darwin is not an appropriate whipping boy for Christians; his insights have been confirmed over the years by a variety of scientific disciplines, and the theory of biological evolution has proven to be indispensable for understanding the world in which we live. Darwin's version of natural selection as the "engine" that has driven evolution may be subject to modification, but there is no question that the concept plays a role in the evolutionary process. I have been critical of two extremes: scientists whose understanding of natural selection would explain the appearance of human beings as purely accidental, and those who insist that scientific evidence clearly demonstrates design and purpose built into the nature of things. There is in this debate middle ground that recognizes both contingency and lawlike structures in the evolution of organic life, making belief in the God of Christian faith an intelligible but not a necessary conclusion. Christians will recognize the awesomeness of creation and the marvel of human life as it has emerged, but they need not and ought not insist that evolutionary biology corroborate their faith by clearly demonstrating that human beings are the goal of the evolutionary process. It is important to remember that while Christian faith is informed and enriched by the results of scientific investigation, particularly as they relate to human existence, faith itself emerges from the breadth and depth of human experience that is not adequately explained by the assumptions of the scientific method.
2. As creatures of evolution, we are in a state of becoming. Human beings are at the far end of a process that began

millions of years ago, and we don't know where it will end. Both as individuals and as a species, we are beings-in-process with a future that is not completely predictable. We might say that *Homo sapiens* is a species that is on a journey that never stops in this life, and journeying involves continuing change. At the present stage of our evolving culture, the changes taking place occur faster than ever before through the impact of developing technologies, a reminder of the "open-endedness" of our existence. As creatures on a journey, we are historical beings whose self-consciousness carries a sense of the past, present, and future. We are the one creature that lives into the future, anticipating what will come and aware of the fact that we are mortal.

3. We are body-selves in relationship, which is a part of our becoming. Our humanity depends upon our being in relationship—with other human beings and the larger creation, all of which is embraced in our relation to God. We find ourselves in finding each other, which is another way of saying that human beings are destined for community and find in community the goal and purpose of their existence. This also means that, by nature, we are moral beings, carrying obligations toward ourselves and toward each other according to our relationships. A powerful gift of the Christian tradition is the capturing of the essence of human relationships and community in the concept of *agapē*, or self-giving love. Rooted in the good news of Jesus Christ as God's Word, this love has the power to generate community and restore the broken relationships that destroy our common life. The one community in which Christians participate that explicitly affirms this agapeic goal is the church, whose task—ongoing but never fully realized—is to embody that goal as well as proclaim it.

4. In light of our biological origins and relatedness to the rest of creation, people of faith can no longer maintain a dualistic view of humanity that identifies our *real* or *essential*

being with a spirit or soul that inhabits a body. We are psychosomatic beings, best understood holistically rather than dividing ourselves into body and soul. What the church historically has understood by "soul" can better be expressed in the concept of our spiritual nature, with reference to the soul understood as a metaphorical expression rather than introducing an ontological dualism. This means that our bodies matter and should not be denigrated in order to elevate our spiritual nature. Just as we do not *have* a soul but *are* spiritual beings, so we do not *have* a body but *are* body-selves, and what we do to our bodies we do to ourselves. It is a severe distortion to understand or treat the body as though it were a machine that can be manipulated with no implications for our spiritual life and sense of identity.

5. Our psychosomatic character also means that any kind of biological reductionism presents an inaccurate, one-sided view of the human being. Genetics and molecular biology provide essential information concerning human nature, but to use their findings as a principle of explanation for the whole realm of human consciousness is to turn the methodology of science into a general epistemology or philosophical position that denies the integrity of our mental and spiritual nature. In challenging this scientific materialism or naturalism, I have made two points that might be characterized as two sides of the same coin: First, the emergence of the human being in biological evolution has constituted a qualitative jump that has created something new, a "bottom-up" movement in the hierarchy of nature that has generated human consciousness and all that it encompasses. Second, there is also a "top-down" movement that recognizes the cultural environment's generative, creative impact on the biological processes of the human organism. The purposive, meaningful nature of conscious human existence is best understood at the macro level of interpersonal relationships rather than through attempts to "explain" that consciousness at the level of microbiology.

6. A distinctive gift of Christian faith is the affirmation that we humans are created in the image of God and thus bear a sacred character that distinguishes us from the rest of God's creatures. However, this uniqueness does not mean a privileged status that removes us from our relations or responsibility to the rest of God's creatures and the natural world. On the contrary, we are thoroughly embedded in God's material world and carry a unique responsibility to it that reflects our standing. The biblical account of creation gives humans "dominion" over God's creation (Gen. 1:28), recognizing our capacity to mold and shape the environment for human ends and purposes. However, for us as moral beings, this dominion constitutes a challenge: it is not an invitation to exploit the environment but to recognize and acknowledge our accountability to God and to each other in the ways we exercise that dominion. Beginning with the Hebrew Scriptures, the biblical witness consistently unites obligations and responsibilities with privileged status.

As we now turn our attention in this and the following chapters to developments in biotechnology, a major part of our discussion will focus on ethical issues. The conclusions summarized here concerning human nature and identity, while providing a basis for an ethical orientation, do not provide specific answers to every question posed by the prospect of human genetic modifications. The Christian churches themselves are divided on what constitutes a proper response to these issues.[1] Some tend to be highly suspicious of any kind of tampering with the human genome, while others are more open to it as long as it serves a life-giving purpose. My discussion in this second part will, I hope, contribute positively to the larger conversation that must continue in the years ahead both in church and in society.

## Defining Biotechnology

The subject of biotechnology, to which we now turn in our consideration of human nature, serves as a particularly forceful reminder of the fact that we live in an evolving culture. I have reflected on our "unfinished" state as human beings, the malleability of human nature and our openness to the future. What this means is that we must become critically aware of the changes posed by biotechnology and the implications they bear for human life and community. It means in particular the need to exhibit a heightened sense of our responsibility as humans in addressing a culture that is increasing our capacity to change ourselves and the environment. Getting a firm grasp on the meaning of both current and potential changes, and discerning the boundary lines that must be drawn to keep them from becoming a threat to our humanity, is a major challenge we face in the years to come.

Technology as the robust offspring of science moves us from the realm of explanation to the realm of engineering, from ideas about our world to actions to change that world. Because knowledge gives us the power to do things, science has led quite naturally to technology. The particular kind of technology we are interested in here, biotechnology, proceeds from the knowledge gained in the biosciences. Forms of biotechnology have actually been around for a long time in such activities as fermentation in the making of bread and cheese and the brewing of wine and beer. Genetic alteration has taken place in animal husbandry through selective breeding, and in agriculture through plant cloning by grafting a shoot or bud onto a growing plant. But these activities would not be regarded as biotechnology in the modern sense.

What is new about modern biotechnology—going back to the mid-1970s—is its manipulation of life forms at the molecular level. The laboratory work required to do this has been tedious and slow, and in no small measure the biotech era has dawned with the arrival of sophisticated tools that not only facilitate this work but have opened up new possibilities. A particularly critical invention was the polymerase chain reaction (PCR), in which computers are used in facilitating the exponential replication of a gene to the numbers needed for laboratory analysis. Through a variety of computers, software programs, automated sequencing machines, fluorescent dyes, lasers, and other machines that have introduced the world of genetic engineering, what had been undreamed of before 1983 became possible. PCR has enabled the analysis of DNA evidence left behind at the scene of a crime and even fragments of DNA from fossils in the remote past. Here is a workable definition:

> "Biotechnology" includes any technique that uses living organisms to make or modify products, to improve plants or animals, or to develop microorganisms for specific uses. Biotechnology has made it possible to expand knowledge about life. It has been used to make new pharmaceuticals, vaccines, and foods; to develop organisms to destroy toxic waste; to make agriculture more productive; to correct genetic defects in humans; and to help stem the destruction of biological diversity.[2]

From this brief definition, one can see that biotechnology covers a lot of ground. It is actually an umbrella term that applies in particular to three major areas of human activity: agriculture, industry, and medicine. Since the 1990s, biotech companies have exerted a huge impact on agriculture through the many uses of genetic engineering. Most crop research focuses on the increase of yields by building in resistance to pests and diseases, tolerance of herbicides, and resilience in the face of drought and other environmental stresses. In livestock industries, the goal is to increase the quantity of animal products, diagnose diseases, and develop vaccines. Reproductive technology, such as cloning, enables farmers to increase the number of offspring from select animals. Genetically modified organisms (GMOs) have become a staple in the human food chain, but not without controversy. Industrial biotechnology is particularly significant in reducing the pollution that comes from an industrialized economy. Since the 1930s, microbes have been used to treat industrial wastewater, and more recently there has been remarkable success in the use of bacteria to clean up oil spills. Since almost everything can be regarded as a food source for one microbe or another, the use of microbes in environmental cleanups has mushroomed. Efforts are now under way to sequence the DNA in entire bacterial communities, with the hope that this effort may lead to engineered microbes that can, among other things, produce hydrogen for fuel and remove carbon dioxide from the atmosphere to help reduce global warming.[3]

The use of biotechnology in medicine, which is our focus here, has created the most intense and controversial moral issues. This is understandable because it involves a move from manipulating objects in our environment to manipulating the cells and organs of our own bodies. The fact that we ourselves have become the objects of technology is nothing new; the medical profession has been working on our bodies since ancient times. What is new, as we have seen, is our vastly expanded knowledge of the human body from the ground up, made possible by genetics and our growing knowledge of the human genome. This knowledge has in turn generated the technology to manipulate and control our bodies at the molecular level. It involves a procedure called "recombinant DNA," in which genes or DNA molecules are spliced and transferred from one source to another, thus modifying organisms by introducing new genes into them. The genius of this procedure is that it mimics what is going on in the natural world, where DNA is constantly transferred into new cellular locations. The procedure can also be done between species because of our common identity at the molecular level; as we have noted, at this level, all creatures speak the same genetic "language." A gene from a bird can be transferred to a fish, or from a pig to a human; it may fail to function in the new organism, but if it does code for a protein, it will carry out the same role in the new organism as it did in the old.

## Developments in Biotechnology

Where medicine traditionally has had the single-minded purpose of healing disease, the application of biotechnology both broadens the scope of healing and opens medical practice to the larger notion of enhancement. These developments are forcing Christians to revisit, in compelling new ways, their understanding of what it means to be human. In contrast to the impact of biological evolution, which turned our attention to the past and the question of human origins, biotechnology focuses our attention on the present and future, raising the question of human destiny. One might expect that, in the coming years, the controversy over biological evolution will gradually subside as Christians come to terms with evolution as "God's way of doing things," but the issues raised by biotechnology are bound to become more intense with the increasing control that biotechnology brings over mind and body.

The major question that society needs to address is "Where are we going with our technology?" or, as we might prefer to put it, "Where is our technology taking us?" and "What is it doing to us as human beings?" We will find that biotechnology is opening new vistas in our understanding of human capacities and our potential for change. That potential is what excites and disturbs the serious observer. Eric Grace's succinct description captures the momentous impact that many are anticipating: "Biotechnology's big promise is to subvert genetic destiny and cure the previously incurable; to rig the lottery and make everyone a winner."[4] At the same time, there is fear that greater control of humans and their environment will quite possibly make everyone a loser. In this section, I note briefly some of the more dramatic developments in biotechnology. All of them raise significant ethical issues, and some in particular raise critical questions about the boundaries of human nature.

It is worth noting at the outset that a significant social consequence of biotechnology is the generation of enormous expectations in the public mind concerning what medicine can accomplish. Genetics appears to be the key that is opening doors to understanding all of our diseases, and that key promises to be the means of conquering them. The growing mastery of medicine in healing our minds and bodies is leading to a subtler shift, where people are inclined to regard themselves, from brains to bones, as a kind of biological machine made up of replaceable or improvable parts. We have noted how the methodology of the biosciences encourages this perspective, in which the human body is analyzed and understood in terms of its parts. Focusing on molecules, cells, and organs becomes the avenue toward understanding the whole. Biotechnology continues and broadens this approach at all levels, from genes to organs, using the tools to successfully manipulate and even to replace those parts of our bodies that are no longer functioning as they should. There have been obvious rewards to this sophisticated technology, but it can also encourage a reductionist understanding of the human body-self that loses sight of our holistic nature.

One of the most fascinating and potentially revolutionary aspects of biotechnology is nanotechnology, which is a spectacular example of biotechnology's focus on life at the molecular level. The prefix *nano-* means "billionth," so a nanosecond is a billionth of a second, and a nanometer is a billionth of a meter (about the length of five to seven atoms, or roughly 100,000th of the thickness of a sheet of paper). Nanotechnology has been defined as "molecules that do things," referring to the use of molecules and even atoms "to create new materials, new processes, and new machines that could improve our lives enormously."[5] A huge step in opening up this technology was the invention in 1990 of the atomic force microscope; it has a needle that can move atoms and molecules around to make new things at a microscopic level. The carbon "nanotube," for example, which is both incredibly strong and light, and nanoparticles are already strengthening and improving any number of items on the market today, including tires and cosmetics.

More remarkable and still in the experimentation stage is the utilization of the power of atoms and molecules to "self-assemble," just as living cells in our bodies do, and then carry out a function designed by human engineers; they literally become little machines. Researchers are pursuing innovative ways to convert the energy generated by the body into electric energy to power nanodevices. Applications include the utilization of the mechanical energy produced by body movement and the hydraulic energy produced by the flow of blood and other bodily fluids. Electrical devices at this nano level—miniature power plants called nanogenerators—would function without the need of batteries and would save a great deal of energy. Researchers see in these developments the potential for revolutionizing the whole realm of electronics. Even viruses and bacteria can be convinced to build devices that are foreign to them, such as semiconductor wires. Applied to medicine, some researchers are working on tiny devices that could travel to a particular organ in a person's body and perform repairs or deliver drugs directly to a cancerous tumor. The one problem that has yet to be solved is whether nanotechnology poses a safety threat. Researchers are concerned about the potential health hazard if nanoparticles were to enter the blood or lungs of factory workers handling these materials. The toxicology of nanoparticles is now being studied, but a big problem is that we haven't yet figured out how to measure the toxicity of something so small.[6]

Assisted reproduction technology (ART) is one of the most publicly recognized areas where biotechnology is already having a profound impact. In England in 1978, Louise Brown was the first baby born from the procedure called in vitro fertilization (IVF); today in the United States alone, more than forty thousand IVF babies are born each year—roughly 1 percent of all live births. IVF involves uniting egg and sperm in a laboratory dish to generate an embryo (what the media call a "test-tube baby"), which is then implanted in a woman's womb to be born nine months later as a healthy child. The procedure was designed for infertile couples, using their gametes (sperm and egg) in order to give them their own biological offspring. This original purpose soon blossomed to include any number of variations, creating what has now become a sizable and prosperous fertility industry. Today, among many options, one can buy eggs and sperm over the Internet, select the sperm of famous people at sperm banks to "upgrade" one's own progeny, freeze eggs for career-oriented women for later impregnation and implantation, arrange for surrogacy in which a woman who is not the biological mother gives birth to the baby, and sort sperm according to the X and Y chromosomes, allowing parents to select a boy or a girl. While most Christian churches have supported the decisions of infertile married couples to use IVF, the entry of the laboratory into "baby making" has resulted in practices and policies that most Christians would regard as at least morally questionable if not theologically unacceptable. The fertility industry is market driven, which means it attempts to come up with a salable product for every conceivable fertility-related need. Ethical questions about the consequences of the industry's policies and products are typically a secondary consideration at best.

It oversimplifies, however, to say that developments in the fertility industry are simply market driven. It is the presence of both the market and the technology that results in reconceptualizing something like infertility so that it is seen as a medical problem that invites medical treatment. In the past, an infertile couple simply faced their infertility as a fact of life with which they must come to terms. They might choose to adopt, but having their own biological children was not an option. The overcoming of this physical obstacle is but one example of a pattern in medical practice where conditions subject to a physician's treatment have dramatically expanded. Achieving greater convenience and expanding the options for living one's life are quite natural imperatives for a consumer society, particularly concerning something as critical to life and health as medicine. Technology is the servant that makes these goals attainable, and for the most part, the submission of technological goals to serious, systematic ethical consideration during the productive process is not likely to happen.[7]

A number of scientists have been particularly enthusiastic in their encouragement of reproductive technology, welcoming the changes it may bring to the mores of society. Gregory Stock, a visiting professor at the University of California, Los Angeles (UCLA), has become particularly notorious for his predictions of what is to come: "With a little marketing by IVF clinics, traditional reproduction may begin to seem antiquated, if not downright irresponsible. One day, people may view sex as essentially recreational, and conception as something best done in the laboratory."[8] Stock's point is that anything that contributes to greater efficiency and control is bound to be desirable to a consumer-driven society. Moving procreation from the bedroom to the laboratory will take the guesswork out of baby making, ensuring the product one desires. This point illustrates well a common attitude among technology visionaries: the market is what determines the mores of the people.

Another significant area of biotechnology is the pharmaceutical industry, which is experiencing a revolution in its production of drugs. Traditionally, drugs have been prescribed on the basis of what works for most people, and because humans are largely indistinguishable in their genetic makeup, most medicines work as intended for all of us. But a difference of a few tenths of 1 percent can be significant when it comes to the effectiveness of a drug. The new science of pharmacogenomics, a combination of pharmacology and genomics, brings a whole new paradigm to the discovery and application of drugs. Our greater knowledge of the human genome enables the pharmaceutical industry to create "designer drugs" that are individualized to go after the causes of a disease as they are expressed in a particular person. In addition, we can better determine which genetic variants lead to adverse, even fatal, reactions that some people have to certain drugs—about a thousand deaths occur each year in the United States from treatments that turn out to be toxic for certain patients.

Another feature of our better understanding of genomics is our increased success in determining genetic variants that predispose a person to a particular disease. Researchers expect that this kind of knowledge will enable the physician to make an accurate prediction concerning the patient's medical future, so preventive measures can be taken well before the onset of disease. DNA testing, for example, is revealing predispositions toward many diseases, such as breast cancer, Huntington's disease, depression, and dementia. The prospect now is to move beyond these tests for a specific disease to assessments of one's total genome. As I write, several companies are beginning to advertise this service at a cost of $1,000, which represents a huge reduction from its initial cost. Using a sampling technique that determines a person's DNA at a million sites along the genome known to vary from person to person, these companies offer a variety of information on one's genotype, including percentage figures on the likelihood of contracting various diseases. However, the fact that the companies make a disclaimer concerning the unqualified accuracy of their findings is a reminder that these genetic tests may be more promise than substance at this point, and they will require more government regulation. Looking further ahead, geneticist Leroy Hood makes an ambitious forecast that promises the virtual elimination of genetic diseases:

> What we'll do is when you're born, we'll take your DNA and look at a hundred disease-predisposing genes, and we'll identify your pattern of predisposition for disease, and then institute appropriate regimes so these things will never come up. Once we're able to do that, we've revolutionized medicine by these preventative techniques. I see this as the real key to gaining control of escalating costs. That's the future and it's very exciting.[9]

## Creating a Superior Human Being

Biotechnology can be put to work not only in overcoming disease and disability, but also in enhancing the condition of people who are functioning within the range of normality. This raises both ethical and theological issues because it appears that we are tampering with human nature itself. The motivation for enhancement comes quite naturally from the desire to succeed, which places us in a competitive relationship with others. One area where competition is particularly focused and intense is professional sports. In recent years, that world has been wracked with turmoil over the use of steroids, human growth hormones, and other stimulants intended to give the athlete an edge over his or her competitors. The competition is so intense, the rewards so substantial in terms of money and prestige, and the drugs so available that it's no surprise that this problem has surfaced. The disseminators of these products that supercharge the athlete's muscles are adept at keeping one step ahead of efforts to regulate and ban them. The reaction of the public for the most part has been quite negative; taking drugs is seen as an unfair advantage, an act that destroys a level playing field and thus constitutes an assault on the integrity of athletic competition.

The sports scene is a kind of microcosm of the larger society, which in many ways appears to be accentuating competitiveness. American life has been characterized as a competitive sport where we jockey intensively for jobs and admission to the most prestigious universities. Building impressive résumés from an early age has become parents' concern for their children. At the same time, competition in society is typically not as focused as it is in organized sports; it is not a matter of taking stimulants in order to win a race or swat a home run. Should we expect of society the same negative attitude that we see in sports toward the use of drugs for enhancement purposes? Are there issues of fairness that come into play here, or is the use of drugs simply a matter of personal privacy and individual responsibility to oneself? The neuroscientist Michael Gazzaniga may reflect a common attitude when he maintains that the enhancement of motor skills would be seen as cheating, but not the enhancement of mental skills. If we can figure out the technology to turn the average Joe into a genius, it just may be the next step in the survival of the fittest. Of people who are fast learners with incredible memories, Gazzaniga observes:

> We accept the fact that they must have some chemical system that is superior to ours, or some neural circuitry that is more efficient. So why should we be upset if the same thing can be achieved by a pill? In some way we were cheated by Mother

Nature if we didn't get the superior memory system, so for us to cheat her back through our own inventiveness seems like a smart thing to do. In my opinion, it is exactly what we *should* do.[10]

At the same time, Gazanniga has some second thoughts about the achievability and possible consequences of this kind of technology: "Having a pill that enhances memory may lead to a whole new set of disorders."[11]

One of the world's chief drivers of human enhancement is the United States military. The Defense Advanced Research Projects Agency (DARPA) funds work along these lines, aimed at a future some twenty to forty years away. In the mid-1980s, DARPA turned its attention to biologically inspired robots, and since the late 1990s, it has increasingly focused on human enhancements, giving a new dimension to the Army slogan "Be All You Can Be." In short, the military is intent on making the soldier as close to unstoppable as possible. This involves creating better, stronger, faster, and smarter human beings. One focus of DARPA's research is to tinker with the internal machinery of human cells in an effort to enhance the soldier's metabolism, leading to greater strength and endurance. Research is being done on sleep deprivation in an effort to create a 24/7 soldier who can function up to a week without sleep. What can we learn from dolphins and whales, who are never fully asleep because they can allow just one portion of their brain to sleep at a time? Research is also being done on expanding available memory space in the brain and developing problem-solving circuits that are sleep resistant. While talk about superhuman strength is avoided, there is interest in cellular research that might increase the efficiency of muscle cells in creating energy, enabling the soldier to function effectively without food as well as sleep for extended periods of time.

A particular focus of DARPA's research is the interface of brain and machine, where thoughts are able to command and control the operation of external devices such as computers. This has tremendous implications for paraplegics and others in the civilian world who are disabled and immobile. If one has an intact central nervous system, a chip can be implanted that enables a measure of external control. Such a chip could also augment brain function and enhance memory, running off the energy in the body. Along the lines of regenerative medicine, one of

DARPA's particularly challenging programs is called Regenesis, which is based on the observation that if you cut off the tail of a tadpole, it will regrow. What prevents this from happening for the adult frog if it loses an appendage? Determining the answer to that question may have implications for humans in possibly regrowing a blown-off hand or in replacing various body parts.[12] The regeneration of organs is, in fact, a promising field today. A team at Wake Forest University has built, from the cell level up, eighteen different types of tissue that include whole organs. Cells have the genetic information necessary to make new tissue, the task being to "direct" them to grow. The goal, already being realized, is to implant these body parts right back into the patients whose cells have been used to make them.[13] Some see the eventual prospect of providing people with their own "banks" of vital organs to use as needed.

Two areas of biotechnology that raise particularly intense ethical and theological issues are genetic enhancement and extension of the human life span. Each of these subjects warrants a fuller discussion (see chapters 5 and 6), but I will briefly introduce them here in spelling out the scope of biomedical technology. Genetic enhancement may not be a realistic prospect anytime soon, but many scientists see it as a reasonable expectation over time. In experiments conducted with chimpanzees and mice, genes have been altered to achieve enhanced performance in problem solving and coping with a variety of challenging conditions, with the assumption that what is being accomplished with these animals can be accomplished among humans as well. Enhancements might include increasing one's height, extending one's life span, and improving one's intelligence. What has happened in recent years to make genetic engineering viable is the combination of reproductive technology, made possible by IVF, with genetics. Bringing human reproduction into the laboratory has not only led to the overcoming of infertility problems, but also opened up the possibility of genetic manipulation of the embryo for both therapeutic and enhancement purposes. This combination of activity inspired Lee M. Silver, a professor of molecular biology at Princeton University, to coin the word *reprogenetics*, which signifies for him a momentous development, not just in the history of science but in the history of humankind:

With reprogenetics, parents can gain complete control over their genetic destiny, with the ability to guide and enhance the characteristics of their children, and their children's children as well.... [It] will turn science fiction into reality, from cloning to embryo selection to genetic engineering, and beyond.[14]

Another part of this scene is reproductive cloning, in which the nucleus of a cell taken from a donor is inserted in an unfertilized egg whose nucleus has been removed, and then the egg is implanted in the womb. The newborn will share the genome of the donor, becoming, in effect, the donor's "delayed twin." While this procedure is successfully performed at the animal level, it is a purely theoretical prospect at the human level. Quite apart from the technical obstacles that would prevent it, society generally and certainly churches find it quite offensive; many states have passed legislation outlawing reproductive cloning, and professional organizations in the scientific community have discouraged their members from pursuing it.

Perhaps the most arresting aspect of biotechnology is what it promises to offer to humankind's perennial search for a fountain of youth. While turning back the aging process is little more than an ardent wish at present, serious efforts now taking place in scientific laboratories around the world promise eventually to extend the human life span significantly. A widely held belief is that nature provides a life span that logically allows for reproducing and raising the young, followed by a natural decline and death. The outside limit for humans now goes well beyond that pattern, with an increasing number of people reaching the century mark and beyond. But for many researchers, present-day figures merely reflect the history of our species up to the present and are not set in stone. They are now focusing on the reasons at the molecular level for bodies to run down and eventually stop, with the goal of slowing down the aging process and perhaps even stopping it or reversing it.[15]

## The Human Machine?

Any thoughtful person reflecting on the present and future impact of biotechnology is likely to be impressed with both its danger and its promise. There are many enthusiastic biotech boosters, including many scientists, who are convinced of its promise and brim with optimism about what it can achieve. However, many other observers see a serious shadow side to biotechnology, worrying about detrimental consequences to human nature and the human psyche, including unintended side effects whose scope and impact are difficult to foresee. Whatever one's expectations about the changes to come, one thing is certain: the rate of change has been accelerating with the development of human culture, and that rate will continue to quicken. Technology has effected such profound changes over such a relatively short time span that our capacity to predict what is to come is more limited than ever. In the past people could look ahead in terms of thirty to fifty years and be fairly confident of what would unfold. Today, however, we no longer have that confidence beyond the next five to ten years. The invention of the computer is a striking example of how technological advance can quickly open up a new future, with an impact that spreads in many different directions. The computer's impact on biology alone has been profound, generating the science of genomics and unlocking the secrets of molecular biology.

Computer power is often expressed in the number of floating-point operations it can execute in a second (abbreviated as FLOPS). IBM in 2005 completed the so-called petacomputer, which is capable of a thousand trillion FLOPS; sometime in the future, there is likely to be a zettacomputer, capable of a billion trillion FLOPS. The brain is thought to have a processing power of one hundred times that of the petacomputer, and it is estimated that by 2015, we will have computers that will equal the processing power of the brain. Contrary to the portrayal of androids in the fantasies of science fiction, however, this does not mean computers will be assuming all the capacities of human beings. They will not be able to function like the brain in terms of human consciousness and experience, but in many respects, they will be far more skilled than the brain. Futurist James Martin speaks of new forms of computer intelligence that he calls "non-human-like" intelligence. Once launched, computers will be able to run under their own steam and improve themselves automatically, "learning" behavior that humans cannot learn, exploring data too vast for humans to explore, and even presenting an evolving behavior that features emergent properties that humans cannot anticipate:

> Ubiquitous machine intelligence that becomes increasingly powerful will be one of the enabling factors that will bring spectacular changes in civilization, but it also sends major alarm signals about whether we can control our technology. Part of the meaning of the 21st century will be learning to coexist with such technology.[16]

Much reflection (and considerable speculation) has been devoted to the prospect that eventually machines will become much more intelligent than humans. Mathematician and computer scientist Vernor Vinge, in his novel *Marooned in Realtime* (1986), borrowed the term *singularity* from astrophysics to describe a time when the curve of technology will become almost vertical and threaten human control. Singularity has since become a common term among many prognosticators, who use it to convey a cataclysmic turn in human history where artificial intelligence exceeds and dominates human intelligence. An explosion of knowledge is anticipated that will surpass the human capacity to understand, setting in motion a chain reaction in computer intelligence and compelling an alliance of human and machine that will bring phenomenal change to all of society. The tight coupling of machine and human intelligence will in turn bring an unprecedented enhancement of human capacities, creating forms of intelligence far more potent than anything we can imagine today. These projections recognize, too, that humans today are using but a small fraction of the brainpower that is available to them. The consequence of these developments will be an immense challenge for humans to summon the ethical and political resources to channel technology in life-serving directions.[17]

A prominent and often controversial exponent of a transformed, technological future is the inventor and futurist Ray Kurzweil. The recipient of many honors in recognition of his inventive genius, Kurzweil sees the singularity kicking in around 2029, by which time we will have fully understood the human brain. That will enable scientists to construct a computer with the hardware capacity of a thousand human brains, far more powerful, faster, and more capable of remembering than the human brain itself. Rather than understanding computer intelligence as "nonhuman," Kurzweil blurs the distinction between human and machine. With singularity, technological change becomes so rapid and so profound that our bodies and brains will merge with our machines. In biblical terms, Kurzweil is promising an eschatological event that will be truly transformative, ushering in a radically new but this-worldly age. In his future world, humans exist who are machine based, whose neurons, flesh, and blood are replaced by electronic and photonic equivalents. Machines will become leading artists, producing creative works. By 2099, he projects, "software-based" humans will number more than the flesh-and-blood types, the result of a physiological and technological evolution in which humans will become "spiritual machines."[18] I believe this kind of speculation is striking proof of the bizarre direction that can result from an anthropology that is based on molecular biology, in this case understanding the human being in terms of the brain's neuronal activity. It is a reductionist view that leads Kurzweil to think that an enhanced human future can be equated with the emergence of high-performing machines.

## Scenarios of the Future

Joel Garreau projects several scenarios or "idea pictures" to help us see the possible results of a world in which biotechnology has changed our bodies and minds.[19] One scenario he terms Heaven, another, Hell, and a third, Prevail—the apocalyptic tone of his language is clearly intended! The Heaven believers are convinced that we are entering a period of exponential change and are impressed with its positive features: increased success in overcoming disease; the enhancement of the human body as it becomes more durable, easier to repair, and more resistant to the aging process; the accomplishment of a unified theory of everything through the achievements of the so-called GRIN technologies (genetics, robotics, information technology, and nanotechnology); and the astonishing enhancement of human capacities and creative abilities ushered in by those technologies. Ideas about human limitations, now culturally entrenched over many years, will be overcome, and a liberated humanity will emerge. What is science fiction today will become reality in a not-too-distant future. Ray Kurzweil would be an obvious example of this point of view.[20]

In stark contrast, while those who believe a Hell lies in our future also are convinced that we face exponential change as a result of technological advances, they are doubtful that we can control those advances for the good of society. For them, the singularity will be a doomsday. The lust for power will be accentuated by the greater control that technology gives us over mind and body; threats to the biosphere will accelerate at an alarming pace; hostilities between tribes, nations, and continents will be exacerbated in the setting of a global village; and we will discover that technology drives history in directions that the rational purposes of human beings cannot restrain or control. This view pictures humans as basically helpless under the onslaught of technologically driven disasters.

The Prevail scenario also recognizes the immense changes and heightened speed of the changes that the future will bring, but it pictures a world in which the good sense and realism of humans will prevail. Those holding to this scenario are impressed with the remarkable ability of humans to muddle through and defy historical forces that appear to be inevitable. Therefore, neither the optimism of the Heaven proponents nor the pessimism of the Hell supporters is warranted. We will be subjected to forces that carry possibilities of both of these scenarios, but the Prevail believers are convinced that ordinary people facing extraordinary odds are capable of rising to the occasion and doing the right thing. Our values can and will shape our future. In this view, technology does not have to determine history; it can be slowed down and diverted in its direction, often in unpredictable ways. An essential aspect of this scenario is the confidence that binding relationships between humans will intensify, and that this heightened sense of social solidarity will provide the basis for overcoming the threats of a highly technologized world.

The critical difference between these scenarios is the measure of human control and direction that each allows in the course taken by technology. The Heaven scenario reveals an unadulterated optimism regarding both the effects of technology and the capacity of humans to direct its course. The Hell scenario is decidedly pessimistic about human efforts to control in any significant way the course taken by technology, believing that technology propels us along as the waves of the ocean carry the swimmer to shore. It develops its own momentum, stimulating wants and desires that refuse to be shut down. The Prevail scenario is willing to bank on human efforts to influence and shape the direction of biotechnology, but not to perfection and not without struggle. It claims a realism that is not found in either of the alternatives, challenging the one extreme of overoptimism, which is blind to the weaknesses of human nature, and the opposite extreme of pessimism, which becomes fatalistic in the face of historical forces, engendering hopelessness in its approach to the future.

A Christian response to these three scenarios summons theological and anthropological convictions that are essential to understanding and evaluating each of them. The Heaven scenario exudes a confidence about the future that the person of faith will regard as highly unrealistic. Its optimism rests on human autonomy and achievement but lacks the tempering influence of a more balanced view of human nature. This scenario reflects naïveté, both in its excessively benign reading of human nature and in its confidence in our capacity to create the world of our fondest dreams. This view recognizes no shadow side to human nature that would be a significant factor in whatever efforts we bring to shaping the world of the future. The reductionist view of human nature will find itself at home in this scenario, because this view's focus on the biological substratum of human life and activity easily ignores the potential for self-centered, destructive actions in the "real world" of human relationships.

The Hell scenario, by contrast, recognizes the shadow side of existence and consequently paints a darker picture of the future world. This reflects a realism familiar to Christian faith, recognizing the pervasive impact of human fallibility and self-centeredness—what we call our sinful nature—on every effort to fashion the future. A careful reading of the past is instructive in this respect, revealing tremendous technological progress in shaping a more livable human existence, but at the same time revealing a world that continues to struggle with inequalities, injustice, poverty, and violence on a worldwide scale. The Hell scenario justifiably asks whether this lack of success and control in the past and present does not pose even greater problems in a future world where the extent of our command and control of our environment and ourselves will be immeasurably enhanced.[21] For the Hell scenario, however, recognizing this fact becomes an invitation to hopelessness because it lacks the confidence that faith inspires. Christian faith carries a profound optimism to its assessment of the future, but its profundity reflects a willingness to recognize the negatives that human nature carries into that future. This means that Christian optimism becomes a tempered optimism, recognizing that every achievement is a mixture of good and bad, strength and weakness, bearing seeds of both threat and promise.

All three of these scenarios of a future biotech world may be far removed from what the future will actually bring. But among the three, I believe that Christian faith would want to affirm the Prevail scenario because it affirms a proper confidence in the capacity of humans to address the future responsibly and to exercise a fitting measure of command over their bodies and the world of nature. That confidence, however, must carry the realism that recognizes our capacity to destroy the kind of future we seek; Christians know better than to think human efforts guarantee a future free of struggle and failure, sickness and death. This would apply in particular to the promise of biotechnology. We want to be open to the creative potential of humanity without denying that we exist within limitations, not all of which can or ought to be transcended. Figuring out those limitations in a way that protects our identity as human beings, affirming the "givenness" of our bodies and minds at the same time that we recognize our "unfinished," evolving character, will demand considerable wisdom and insight on the part of both church and society.

## Concluding Thoughts

A critical question at the outset of any consideration of biotechnology, and one that has been much discussed, is whether biotechnology hasn't attracted so much hype and overstatement as to make extremely difficult any effort to reach an astute and accurate judgment on what it will actually mean for human nature and the human future. The onset of any new technological era in the past—such as the emergence of the atomic age, for example—has excited many expressions of cataclysmic change that with the passing years can look quite overdrawn and wide of the mark. Perhaps this is the case with biotechnology. We do need to maintain perspective, seeing the continuities with the past of any new breakthrough in technology and not succumbing to the excitement and exaggerated claims that such developments are bound to create. But this point can also be misused. For example, one could have greeted the advent of the airplane as simply a logical progression in the mode of travel going back to ancient times, moving a body from one point to another. That judgment would have missed the larger truth that the airplane (and subsequently the jet engine that powers it) signaled a huge, transformative impact, not just on transportation but in helping to create a new and much smaller world with vast new possibilities for human interaction.

In the light of medical practice, the tools used by an emerging biotechnology could be seen, too, as simple extensions of medical technology, but this view would not capture the meaning of biotechnology. I have noted its roots in the investigations of the biosciences that have uncovered the secrets of cellular life, introducing a paradigm jump in understanding who and what we are. What makes biotechnology distinctive is its capacity to manipulate the human organism at this micro level, tinkering with the genetic material essential to our humanity. The human body has thus become an object in a new way, subject to manipulation and change at a fundamental level that can threaten our sense of who we are as human beings. Much of the current controversy over this development is between those who are deeply concerned about its implications for our understanding of human nature and those who believe we are witnessing a natural progression in the evolution of the human species. Among the latter group are those who would claim we have good reason to celebrate any change that promises greater mastery of the environment, and that should include the enhancement of human capacities.

An appropriate ethical response to biotechnology has been a lively issue among Christian bioethicists, creating significant divisions that are often characterized on the basis of ideology—either conservative or liberal perspectives. Gilbert Meilaender at Valparaiso University takes the discipline of bioethics to task for failing to give sufficient attention to the meaning of being human, rightly noting the challenge that biotechnology represents to our understanding of humanity. He advocates a more principled approach that would set definite limits to avoid potentially harmful developments in biotechnology, resulting in an unambiguous "Go no further," instead of the anemic "Proceed with caution" that is too often heard.[22] The problem is that many of these issues are not clear-cut, compelling one to balance competing values that defy a categorical response. While I appreciate the concerns expressed by ethicists like Meilaender—concerns that have prompted the writing of this book—there is still room for differing perspectives on where to draw the line in challenging the excesses of biotechnology. It is typical of conservative voices in this debate to draw the line at embryonic stem cell research or even the use of in vitro fertilization, a stance that I believe is not ethically warranted. But the issues are serious enough to compel an honest effort among bioethicists to find common ground in staking out an ethical position.

A major reason for the hype surrounding biotechnology is the claim that it promises the eventual elimination of genetic diseases. The possibility is exciting but should also provoke some second thoughts. In the dynamic world of living things, we do not know what is coming around the corner in the form of another problem or threat to our well-being, nor do we know whether a solution to one problem won't create a new and possibly worse problem for the next generation. We also cannot afford to forget the far less glamorous reality that low-tech, preventive measures involving self-discipline and responsible effort will always be essential to the achievement of health and well-being. As Eric Grace observes, "Expensive, sophisticated, high-tech medicine does not guarantee longer, healthier lives any more than expensive, sophisticated high-tech weapons guarantee world peace."[23] Rather than conquering disease, the outcome of biomedical technology could be that it saves some individuals from some diseases while the majority of our citizens have little or no access to it. This is a reminder of the fact that politics and economics play as important a role as the technology itself if its promise is to be realized in any significant way.

Much has been said of "the technological imperative." For biotechnology, that imperative involves such factors as the promise it excites in combating diseases and promoting human health and well-being, the fascination with microbiology that continues to unveil secrets about our biological nature, and the powerful appeal of success itself, enhanced by continuing reports of new and surprising achievements in scientific laboratories around the world. All of these factors contribute to euphoria over what technology can accomplish, and we can understand the grandiose visions it has inspired. In spite of the promise, however, biotechnology is in many respects a two-edged sword. Its very success has generated a variety of ethical questions and dilemmas, including uncertainty about its long-term impact on the culture and mores of society. What human costs are involved in the quest for greater convenience and a more pleasurable life that characterizes the drive of technology? The imperative to ease the more onerous burdens of human existence, admirable in itself, raises the question of human limits and whether the fact that we *can* do something is sufficient reason to believe that we *ought* to do it. The gravity of these issues demands a serious effort on the part of churches to address them and to make their voice heard in the public discussion of these matters.

From a theological perspective, the euphoria over technological advances becomes an expression of idolatry when it hails technology as a final answer to the human predicament, a solution to all that plagues and thwarts the flourishing of humanity. This is to define the human predicament in terms that technology can solve, which for the Christian is a profound misreading of the richness and complexity of human life. As a human endeavor, biotechnology will always remain subject to abuse, with the greater capacity to enhance human traits and qualities accompanied by the excesses of ambitions and desires that know no limits. The continuing challenge, both personal and political, is to bring a degree of wisdom and insight to the use of technology that enables society to utilize it in achieving a more just and humane community. Technology in all its forms can significantly improve the conditions in which we live out our lives, but it cannot save us from ourselves. This is a reality that we must not overlook in the face of proposals to improve or enhance what it means to be human.

CHAPTER 5

# HUMAN NATURE AND GENETIC ENGINEERING

T he previous chapter's discussion of biotechnology included brief mention of what we call genetic engineering (GE). In this chapter, I want to examine more closely the meaning of GE and the implications it poses for our understanding of human nature. The term is revolutionary, moving genetics in a dramatic way from *studying* the heritable traits of human beings to *modifying* those traits. In other words, it is genetics united with technology in order to effect changes in the human body that are seen as necessary or desirable. This movement is captured by another expression one often hears, the "new genetics." What is new is this uniting of the science of genetics with technology, most often with the purpose of treating a diseased patient but also introducing the possibility of improving the capacities and performance of human beings. The Human Genome Project has made the new genetics possible, opening up the science of genomics and giving a powerful stimulus to GE. While GE has long taken place in laboratories, where scientists work on many forms of life from bacteria to mice, and while the world of agriculture has long profited from GE in the manipulation of animals and crops, it is only in more recent years that serious attention has been given to the engineering of the human genome.

## What Is Genetic Engineering?

Genetic engineering is customarily divided into two kinds, somatic and germinal. Somatic GE (from the Greek word *soma*, meaning "body") refers to modification of genetic material in the body cells of an individual. This is accomplished by a procedure called gene transfer in which a gene is added to or replaces a gene in the tissue or an organ of an individual, and the effects of the transfer are limited to that individual. Germinal GE is applied to an individual's gametes or sexual cells (sperm or eggs), which means that the effects of the modification are transmitted to everyone in the generations that follow. This would be a more efficient procedure, because it would be a onetime course of action that would not have to be repeated, as with somatic GE. Because of its extensive impact and possibly negative consequences, the prospect of germinal GE also raises more serious issues for medical practice and ethics. While *germinal GE* or *germ line therapy* has been the common terminology, a more comprehensive and adequate expression recommended by the American Association for the Advancement of Science is *inheritable genetic modifications*, which refers to "any biomedical intervention that can be expected to modify the genome that a person can transfer to his or her offspring."[1] Besides the direct altering of egg and sperm, this would include the use of other technologies now under development, such as cellular surgery and the insertion of artificial chromosomes into the embryo in an effort to overcome some of the obstacles associated with single-gene transfer. Artificial chromosomes would add a "gene-pack" of hundreds or thousands of new genes and would ensure a more successful passage for them into the embryo.[2]

As we have noted, the driving interest in GE as it relates to medicine is the prospect of curing or preventing diseases at the molecular level; gene transfer is aimed at defective genes that are the culprit in causing genetic disease. The task is to transfer a normal copy of the defective gene into the affected cell, with the hope that the addition of a corrective gene will compensate for the defective one. If it does, the vital protein that is lacking will be produced again, and that protein will act as a therapeutic agent. The success of this procedure is most promising where a disease can be traced to the abnormality of a single gene, including such diseases as Huntington's, cystic fibrosis, Tay-Sachs, and sickle-cell anemia, among the roughly twelve hundred disorders that geneticists associate with a single gene. The gene can either be transferred in the laboratory, where cells are taken from the patient and genetically altered, or be injected directly into the body cells of the patient. A virus is typically used as a vector or carrier, bringing the gene to the diseased cell and injecting it. Normally, this would mean the virus is infecting the cell, but because it has been treated, the action is not pathogenic; the virus is incapable of replicating itself.

While this description may seem relatively straightforward, the process is actually highly complicated and risky for several reasons, including potential problems with viral carriers and the considerable challenge of getting the gene to properly integrate into the recipient genome and then getting it to function correctly. The modified gene has to become active in precisely the right place, at the right time, and to the right extent. Accurately identifying the target cell and achieving efficient delivery methods also are formidable challenges. There are other obstacles as well, such as the short life of the introduced gene and the response of the body's immune system; repeated rounds of therapy may be needed. These obstacles have prevented gene modification from becoming an available procedure at the clinical level. For example, the muscular dystrophy gene was identified in 1983, but we are still unable to apply the needed therapy. At this point, it is fair to say that gene modification is too susceptible to uncertainty and error to make it a viable option for human beings.[3] The use of the term *gene therapy* is now generally discouraged, because it can give the public the impression that genetic cures are now fully available or at least are just around the corner. This is not the case.

My discussion of DNA in chapter 3 points to still further problems for GE and the prospect of gene therapy. We have learned that there are many variables in our understanding of genes, including cellular activity and the influence of the environment. We cannot assume that there is a direct line from the gene to its expression at the level of human behavior or even in regard to the presence of a genetic disease. To be sure, the connection between a certain gene and a particular genetic disease can be reasonably clear, but even here, any prediction of what will occur for a particular individual is subject to many factors besides genetics. Toxic elements in the environment, diet, drugs, climate, and lifestyle can all play a role. Moving from the molecular level to bodily life in society—from genotype to phenotype—is thus no simple matter, whatever the condition one is addressing. Nonetheless, in spite of all the technical challenges and the inherent ambiguities in understanding gene expression, the potential benefits of gene modification appear to be so great that most people are inclined to support continuing efforts to make it a useful weapon in combating disease. There is always reason to be hopeful, but one must guard against exaggerated expectations concerning what gene modification will ultimately accomplish.

There are other, less invasive means than GE of contending with genetic diseases, and they are being increasingly used. Genetic screening and testing have become widespread, particularly where individuals have a family history of genetic disease. This has led to the practice of preimplantation genetic diagnosis (PGD), where in vitro fertilization technology is used to examine embryos in the laboratory for defective genes prior to implantation in the womb. This allows for embryo selection, where diseased embryos are discarded and a healthy embryo implanted. It also allows for sex selection and the prospect of other kinds of enhancement decisions, raising obvious ethical concerns. Another procedure, now greatly improved as a result of the completed mapping of the human genome, is preimplantation genetic screening (PGS), where both parents-to-be and fetuses are screened for genetic diseases. If the fetus is diseased, the tragic choice facing the parents is abortion. To make this choice in the case of a devastating disease is understandable, but screening has also raised a secondary question that is still more unsettling: Is abortion an acceptable option if the fetus does not bear a defective gene but is a *carrier* of that gene? The fact that this question is posed at all is troubling evidence of what happens with increased mastery and control of our bodies, including the reproductive process. It fuels a drive for perfection, or in this case the removal of every possibility of disease.

The increased use of prenatal screening has prompted some concern about the cultural impact of such a practice. The fear is that, instead of unconditional acceptance of the newborn, it may encourage an attitude of conditional acceptance based on the presence of desirable traits. The question is whether this form of negative eugenics, where we abort a fetus that is unacceptable because of a genetic disease, is but a small step from insisting on criteria for an acceptable fetus. Could we be on the way to subjecting birth to a form of "quality control" that ensures parents of a desirable "product"? Too much can be made of the slippery-slope argument, but it can be a healthy reminder in this case that a concern to get rid of negative features in the newborn can run the danger of insisting on positive features as the prerequisite to acceptance of him or her. This attitude was quite plain in a question asked by a parent who had selected a sperm donor with "high intelligence" to be the biological father of his child: "Why is it OK for people to choose the best house, the best schools, the best car, but not try to have the best baby possible?"[4] This gentleman is obviously receptive to genetic enhancement, should the opportunity become available.

## From Therapy to Enhancement

In considering human nature—the "Who are we?" question—the subject of genetic enhancement raises the most serious issues. While there are Christians who would reject any kind of genetic manipulation as an improper intrusion on the body that God has given us, many would likely find the prospect of genetic therapy an acceptable goal but draw the line at efforts to enhance or improve upon a person's physical and mental capacities. To draw the line between therapy and enhancement, however, is challenging. Many would argue that it defies being done because there is no evident line between the two. It involves the definition of health or normal functioning, but these concepts lie in the eye of the beholder; what appears to be in the range of normal health to one person is regarded as a health problem or disability to another. In recent years, the World Health Organization has redefined its understanding of health in terms of a sense of general well-being, rather than the absence of disease, a definition that encourages a fair amount of disagreement over what constitutes health, because of the nebulousness of "well-being." One's understanding of health is also shaped by one's individual circumstances; the presence of color blindness, for example, may strike most of us as within the range of normalcy, but to one who aspires to be an airline pilot, it is a serious defect. If shortness of stature—not just dwarfism, but measuring a few inches below the statistical average—disturbs the mental well-being of a person, she may well regard herself as subnormal and in need of help if it is available.

Difficult as it may be to distinguish between genetic modification as therapy or enhancement, the distinction is important and needs to be made. For the most part, there is little difficulty in distinguishing the two. Any genetic disease that disables and finally destroys a person is clearly a candidate for therapy and has nothing to do with enhancement as we are discussing it here. (One could say that curing a person's disease is a form of enhancement, but that is a different use of the term.) Assuming it can be done by genetic modification, improving the intelligence quotient of a child from the rating of average to near genius, or increasing his height from a projected six feet to seven feet, is clearly enhancement, not therapy. When we move from these extremes of curing devastating disease versus inducing dramatic enhancements to the much larger middle realm of disabilities, it becomes more difficult to make the distinction between therapy and enhancement. At this point, our judgments become value laden, reflecting social and personal attitudes that play a role in shaping one's perspective on what constitutes a disability. This fact would suggest that if genetic therapy is to become a weapon in the arsenal of the medical profession, it should receive validation and support from government only in regard to the amelioration or elimination of life-threatening diseases. Where our compassion is most deeply moved by the plight of our fellow humans, there the radical intrusion of genetic treatment would be justified.

Having made this point, however, one must acknowledge its theoretical character. As noted, gene therapy is still far removed from clinical practice, with many obstacles yet to be overcome. To be sure, there have been some notable successes,[5] but they do not signify a breakthrough in the treatment of genetic disease. It is important, nonetheless, to consider well in advance under what conditions somatic and germ line therapy could be utilized. Given the far more extensive impact of germ line modification and the greater seriousness of any unforeseen consequences, there is generally more willingness to consider somatic gene treatment. The following criteria have been proposed as requirements to govern human germ line modification should it become feasible:

- there are no other treatments available;
- it has been proven effective or at least more effective than other therapies;
- its potential benefits for the patient outweigh the risks;
- it inflicts less pain or suffering than other forms of treatment.[6]

To require all four of these conditions is setting the bar quite high, but that is where it should be when we are dealing with medical activity involving inheritable genetic modifications. Altering the genome as a method of therapy is so unlike other types of medical therapy that it severely challenges our ability to estimate potential harms. If we ever come to the point where the four criteria are met, and assuming adequate regulation that limits treatment to catastrophic diseases, I would be in favor of germ line modification because of the widespread healing impact it promises for generations to come. This means that I do not regard DNA as a sacred realm that ought never to be altered. It all depends on the purpose and goal of such action. Healing a catastrophic disease would justify this kind of medical intrusion.

Admittedly, to limit GE to a therapeutic use in a society like ours would be a challenge. Social conditions play a role in this matter, and in an affluent, consumer society like ours, the drive for enhancement of every conceivable kind is both intense and widespread. This fact is dramatically apparent in the area of psychopharmacology, where antidepressants are widely used as mental enhancers among people who hardly qualify as depressed. "Almost 38 million people in the world today are prescribed Prozac, and at least as many are taking some closely related drug. . . . The reality is that Prozac and its clones affect both the depressed and the nondepressed."[7] Another example of blurring the line is the antidepressant drug Paxil, which has been found to reduce anger in nondepressed individuals and make them more socially adept. Ritalin is widely used for both medical and nonmedical purposes, prescribed for attention deficit/hyperactivity disorder (ADHD) but commonly used as a stimulant by college students to enhance their performance on exams. Considerable pressure is exerted by pharmaceutical companies to enlarge the range of conditions that call for their products, encouraging people to "medicalize" their problems and find handy solutions in the form of a pill. Some predict that an increasing amount of medical practice will be nontherapeutic, designed to enhance normal human capacities rather than to cure diseases.

Cosmetic surgery is another common form of enhancement in the United States. In 2002 some $7 billion was spent on noncorrective cosmetic surgery; a case in point would be the 350,000 nontherapeutic breast augmentations that occurred that year. In 2003 Americans underwent 1.8 million plastic surgeries, up from 330,000 a decade earlier. In 2004 the American Society for Aesthetic Plastic Surgery issued suggestions for "improving quality of life" for every stage of adult life: Botox injections with a tummy tuck and breast lift in the thirties following childbirth; lipoplasty for double chin and fat deposits in the forties; a facelift, eyelid surgery, and lip augmentation in the fifties; and more Botox, skin resurfacing, fat injections, and repeat facelift in the sixties.[8] We are used to regarding our bodies as objects that can be improved and enhanced in a multitude of ways, which likely means we are more than ready for the advent of genetic enhancements.

Some would suggest that the use of drugs and surgery provides a precedent that would justify genetic enhancement, but I believe that altering a person's genome for enhancement purposes is a qualitatively different action from taking drugs to modify behavior or submitting to surgery to improve one's appearance. Apart from the level of intrusion being much more profound, enhancement represents an attempt to recreate oneself with a new genetic identity that endows uniquely new potential. Another factor in this scene is the increased expectations that people bring to medicine in light of its dramatic progress over the past century. The very success of medicine cultivates a desire for more services and the conquering of new frontiers. And of course the more affluent a society, the more ready it is to indulge in anything that promises to improve one's appearance and performance.[9]

One area where the pressure to use GE for enhancement purposes could be particularly strong is in the parent-child relationship. We live in an age of hyperparenting, where parents will go to any length to see their children, from preschool toddlers to college students, excel. If genetic enhancements were available, many would regard failure to pursue them as a dereliction of duty. Much of the same dynamic that we noted in the previous chapter concerning athletics is present here; people are always interested in gaining the competitive edge, particularly for their children. Should genetic enhancement become widespread, children would increasingly become the picture of what their society values in terms of appearance and abilities. What is "normal" as perceived by the majority population would ultimately prevail, leading to greater homogeneity within the society. "In essence, we and our children increasingly will be reflections of our personal philosophies and values. Where today we sculpt our minds and bodies using exercise, drugs, and surgery, tomorrow we will also use the tools that biotechnology provides."[10] What this would amount to is a eugenics program, not dictated by government but driven "from the ground up" by the choice of parents who have the power to control the kind of offspring they desire.

## The Enhancement Argument

In following the debate over GE for the purpose of human enhancement, one can discern roughly three groups of people in the positions taken. One group consists of optimists concerning the future course of biotechnology; they see genetic enhancements as a natural and inevitable progression in the evolving nature of human beings. Another group consists of those who are not opposed on grounds of principle to genetic enhancements, but they are wary of some serious obstacles that lie in the way. These may be technical obstacles that members of this middle ground believe will not be overcome, or political and economic obstacles that will prevent many from gaining access to genetic enhancements, posing a substantial social justice issue. The final group consists of those who are opposed to enhancement on grounds of principle; on philosophical or theological grounds, they believe any attempt to genetically change the boundaries of our nature is both wrong and irresponsible, and may also carry unintended consequences that society will deeply regret. In this section, I will focus on the arguments of the first group in favor of genetic enhancements.

The prospect of altering genes in order to enhance one's intellect, memory, moods, and other personal traits will likely impress most people as preposterous, and with good reason. Our capacity to effect such changes in humans is still far from being realized, and the social and political resistance to attempting it would be substantial. Indeed, many scientists regard genetic enhancement as little more than science fiction and not worth serious attention. Nonetheless, some members of the scientific community insist that what is being accomplished in genetic experimentation with animals is the prelude to serious efforts at enhancing human capacities and performance. This belief is supported by their understanding of what it means to be human. A notable exponent of enhancement medicine, Gregory Stock, sees the emergence of GE and the prospect of germ line therapy and germ line enhancement—what he calls "germinal choice technology"—as a natural development in the train of human evolution that has been building over thousands of years:

> The arrival of germinal choice technology signals a diffuse and unplanned project to redesign ourselves. But it is neither an invasion of the inhuman, threatening that which is human within us, nor a transcendence of our human limits. Remaking ourselves is the ultimate expression and realization of our humanity. . . . We are beginning an extraordinary adventure that we cannot avoid, because, judging from our past, whether we like it or not this *is* the human destiny.[11]

This conviction of Stock is linked with considerable optimism concerning the ability of researchers to overcome the technical difficulties that stand in the way of germinal choice technologies. "Pure and simple, we are poised to make conscious, highly specific choices about the genetic constitutions of our children and to inject our preferences into the next generation using methods far beyond those previously available."[12] Stock welcomes the increase in genetic screening in order to avoid diseases "and other unwanted traits," and believes this desire to exclude negatives in human existence will continue quite logically with efforts to accentuate the positive through genetic enhancements. It is true that with ongoing development of ever more sophisticated screening techniques, researchers may be able to detect genetic markers that correlate statistically with certain desirable traits such as tallness, leanness, perfect pitch, longevity, and perhaps temperament and even intelligence.[13] But contrary to Stock's optimism, this knowledge is far from enabling us to alter these traits through genetic manipulation. One can imagine, should this kind of engineering ever be realized, that Congress would likely pass laws to make it illegal, a prospect that does not impress Stock. If clinical trials are prevented in the United States, they will occur "in government labs in China, or in clandestine facilities in the Caribbean."[14] The power of self-directed evolution is too great to be stopped by government intervention.

Stock recognizes the validity of the argument that the safety of people should be our paramount concern, and he acknowledges that science is not yet ready to do the experimenting with humans that would be required to successfully arrive at germ line enhancement. That may still be the case a decade from now, too, but he anticipates that the story will be different two or three decades from now. Time is a factor today but not indefinitely; the real issue, Stock says, is philosophical and religious beliefs. "It is about what it means to be human, about our vision of the human future."[15] That vision for Stock appears to have no bounds; he speaks of reaching the point "at which we may be able to transform ourselves into something 'other.'" What that provocative language means, however, is not clear, for he goes on to say, "We cannot know where self-directed evolution will take us, nor hope to control the process for very long."[16] In other words, who we will become depends on the nature of future technologies and the kinds of values that will emerge in the human future, both of which we cannot now see or comprehend. What is sure is that the evolutionary trajectory thus far promises a future in which human beings are sufficiently transformed to become a species distinct from *Homo sapiens*. For enhancement advocates, that kind of development lies well within the limits of what it means to be human.

A common conviction in the advocacy stance is that the dynamics of the market system should shape the course of this technology.

It is a ground-up phenomenon, fueled by the wants and desires of the population and particularly of parents who seek the very best for their children. It seems to be assumed that if a particular trait or talent is a want or desire of parents for their children, it is justified. "If we could make our baby smarter, more attractive, a better athlete or musician, or keep him or her from being overweight, why wouldn't we?"[17] Parents bear responsibility for their children on any decision relating to their future well-being, and as Lloyd Cohen observes, this calls for a laissez-faire approach: "As a general matter, we trust parents to make decisions that affect the future health, character, and personality of their children. I can see nothing substantially different in the case of germ line engineering that warrants a different policy."[18] This comment also brings out another feature typical of enhancement arguments: they see no qualitative difference between genetic enhancements and any other effort at self-improvement. A comment by John Harris, which would strike many people as a wild non sequitur, reflects this point: "And if . . . it is not wrong to attempt to improve something like intelligence by education, why should it be wrong to attempt to improve it by genetic manipulation?"[19] This is a kind of utilitarian thinking that seems incapable of distinguishing between the means that are used to achieve the end; not every means is justified by the end.

The visionary character of much advocacy of enhancement strikes one as utopian. What biomedicine will be able to achieve appears to be limitless, creating new human beings whose future promises everything they could desire. An example of this kind of thinking is found quite prominently in Gregory Pence, a physician and professor at the University of Alabama School of Medicine, who projects for future generations "a body free of the dangerous genetic diseases, a body that can function well for at least a hundred years, intelligence and good memory, and a personality that is disposed to be happy. Life is better when it starts this way."[20] These dreams of a new human being are often reflected in the titles of books written by advocates, such as Lee Silver's *Remaking Eden* (1997), Gregory Stock's *Redesigning Humans* (2003), and Ramez Naam's *More Than Human* (2005). Their enthusiasm for the prospects of change is not dampened by resistance, which they see variously as lack of courage, knowledge, and vision. They are also convinced that while every technological innovation applied to the human body generates initial opposition, that opposition is gradually overcome. The following observation concerning assisted reproductive technology would, they believe, be applicable to GE as well:

> Any change in custom or practice in this emotionally charged area has always elicited a response from established custom and law of horrified negation at first; then negation without horror; then slow and gradual curiosity, study, evaluation, and finally a very slow but steady acceptance.[21]

Impatience with the resistance of society and the medical establishment in particular is directed by Gregory Pence at the "backward looking, overly cautious medical ethics" of professionals in medicine, who have stymied progress over the years in such areas as the treatment of infertility, stem cell research, and the donation of organs. He maintains that the notion of "natural limits" is invalid and functions as a roadblock to medical progress, which he believes should include the prospect of parents choosing the genetic traits of their children.[22] The guiding question, says Pence, is "What's in the best interest of the people to come?" He has no doubt that genetic enhancements will result in a much better, more humane world. In an imaginary letter projected for 2010, written to generations yet to come, he writes, "How can we *not* try to improve your lives?" He sees all concerns being raised today as trumped by the anticipated progress made possible by GE and pharmacology, resulting in the enhancement of memory, intelligence, and learning as well as solving the problem of obesity, to say nothing of countering genetic diseases like cystic fibrosis.[23] Pence lumps all potential uses of GE together, making a moral argument on behalf of both therapy and enhancement that ignores any reason to distinguish between them.

## The Anti-enhancement Argument

People who bring serious reservations to the subject of genetic enhancements express a variety of concerns: doubts about the ability to overcome the technical demands, concerns about securing the safety of patients, fears about unintended consequences that would affect generations to come, philosophical reasoning that questions the underlying assumptions of the quest for enhancements, ethical concerns about the injustices likely to result in a gene-centered society, and theological reservations about "playing God" and threatening the very concept of human nature. My critique here will focus primarily on the last three—philosophical, ethical, and theological concerns.

## *The "Genocentric" Fallacy*

One thing that impresses the observer is the remarkable confidence and breathtaking expectations that some scientists bring to the prospect of genetic enhancements. This is all the more remarkable in view of the fact that, at this point, the prospect is far from being realized. Virtually everything is a matter of anticipation, and what fuels it is the philosophical conviction that genetics is revealing an ultimate picture of the human being—a revelation, if you will—that for the first time gives humanity a glimpse of its destiny. However, this is not science but ideology, and fortunately, scientists themselves are among its most forceful critics. The evolutionary biologist Richard Lewontin, whom we have met in previous chapters, brings a trenchant critique:

> The last fifty years have seen the reorganization of most biology around DNA as the central molecule of heredity, development, cell function and evolution. Nor is this reorganization only a reorientation of experiment. It informs the entire structure of explanation of living processes and has become the center of the general narrative of life and its evolution. An entire ideology has been created in which DNA is the "Secret of Life," the "Master Molecule," the "Holy Grail" of biology, a narrative in which we are "lumbering robots created, body and mind" by our DNA. This ideology has implications, not only for our understanding of biology, but for our attempts to manipulate and control biological processes in the interests of human health and welfare, and for the situation of the rest of the living world.[24]

One implication of Lewontin's comment is that the prospect of GE ought not to be seen as a necessary "next step" in the course of medical progress, and certainly not as a final climax to that progress. Its appeal as a high-tech solution to medical problems should be understood as reflecting a gene-centered or genocentric mind-set, justifying and encouraging genetic intrusion as the ultimate way of solving those problems. The ideological factor he mentions has already gained our attention in the first three chapters in the form of sociobiology and scientific materialism, and now Lewontin is saying that with GE, we see a consequence of the determinist thinking that characterizes those views. I do not believe that this means human GE, including efforts at gene therapy, has to be repudiated across the board, but it does mean that its prominence on the medical horizon requires some hard, critical thinking that raises philosophical as well as medical questions. One can be open to its genuine promise without jumping on its bandwagon; we are best served by looking critically at every facet connected with the practice and potential of GE, rather than by greeting it as a knight in shining armor.

The genocentric view of human beings has widespread implications for medical practice. For example, my earlier reference to genetic screening assumes a hierarchy of causes in the occurrence of disease, with genes at the very top. This is justified in contexts where a particular genetic disease is clearly indicated from the patient's family history. But where screening becomes common practice, there is clearly the risk that a genocentric ideology is ruling medical practice. Biologist Ruth Hubbard is another scientist who is sensitive to the impact of genocentrism, seeing its consequences well beyond genetic testing:

> We urgently need to demedicalize our relationship to our bodies and our state of health. . . . Our new fixation on genes can only make us less confident about our bodily functioning and so increase our alienation from ourselves. We need to engage in active debates about the practical consequences of genetic forecasts for our self-image, our health, our work lives, our social relationships, and our privacy.[25]

These statements of Lewontin and Hubbard make a significant point about human nature that is particularly meaningful because it is made by biologists who are intimately familiar with the methods and assumptions that lead to the genocentric perspective. We can infer from their critique that an adequate understanding of the human being cannot be gained from what goes on at the microscopic level; who we are must be approached from the macro world of human relationships and self-awareness.

The truth of this point is driven home by attempts to understand and manipulate a trait such as intelligence, which would be an obvious choice for genetic enhancement. A genocentric view assumes that intelligence can be enhanced through GE, but without really coming to grips with what this would mean from the personal perspective of the individual. We are still far from knowing all the genes that play into a polygenic trait such as intelligence, but even if we did know, it is hardly possible to predict how altering any of these contributing genes would affect one's intelligence. The effect of any genetic alteration would not likely be limited to a particular gene; one would have to be concerned about the effect on other parts of the person's personality as well, which could be incalculable. David Resnick makes the further observation, "When a person's unpredictable life experience is then thrown into the equation, the number of possible outcomes is infinite. Although it is conceivable that a trait such as intelligence could selectively be altered, it is impossible to predict how such an alteration would truly affect a person's life, positively or negatively."[26]

These observations bring us back to the truth we've noted in earlier chapters: human beings can be understood only within a holistic perspective that moves us well beyond our genes. Whether speaking of enhancement or the treatment of disease, one cannot avoid the fact that our genetic constitution is embedded in a network of biological and ecological relationships that have an effect on the way our genes operate. This fact was dramatized some years ago when the same gene was inserted in a mouse embryo and a hog embryo with opposite effects: the mouse grew to twice its normal size, and the hog became leaner than normal. The way the gene functioned "depended on other things going on in the organism.... Molecular biologists emphasize the role of genes in this situation because they are more interested in genes than in the development of mice or hogs.... In very few cases can a gene legitimately be said to be 'for' any one thing."[27]

The Human Genome Project, which caught the imagination of the public during the last decade of the twentieth century, has contributed significantly to a cultural environment that is focused on the gene as a primary source for understanding human nature. Back in the mid twentieth century, social scientists were inclined to believe that culture and environment were decisive in accounting for variance in human behavior. The behaviorist school had its various representatives—notably B. F. Skinner—but they were far from being a majority at the time. Then came the rise of disciplines like behavioral genetics and evolutionary psychology, and the tide began to change. Our culture "has become infatuated with human genetics. Where we used to look for environmental causes we now look for genetic ones. We ignore mountains (the environment) in order to focus on molehills (genes)."[28] The laboratory is now regarded as the primary source for new insights into human nature, as virtually every week a new discovery is reported that sheds light on human biology and behavior. With the rise of biotechnology, the prospect of human and social engineering has taken on a high profile, with the implication that humans are essentially biological machines reducible to their chemical and biological components. We are encouraged to believe that the geneticist and molecular biologist now have the keys not only to healing the diseases that plague humanity but also to shaping and predicting the future course that humanity will take. The genetic ideology has become a pervasive cultural phenomenon.

## Ethics and Human Fulfillment

The genetic ideology has significant implications for ethics and our understanding of human fulfillment. A notable expression of this ideology is found in Richard Dawkins's *The Selfish Gene*, which in its own way makes its contribution to the attraction of genetic enhancements. In a world of competition, we seek an edge over our neighbor, and if our personal abilities and gifts are due to our genes, then genetic enhancement is the ultimate solution to getting ahead. The depiction of life in Dawkins's book is one of ruthless competition that is justified by our gene-driven nature: "We, and all other animals, are machines created by our genes.... A predominant quality to be expected in a successful gene is ruthless selfishness."[29] Dawkins assures us that he is not advocating an ethics of selfish behavior, but his characterization of human beings as gene machines not only invites gene enhancement as the avenue to success, but also accentuates the individual in isolation from his or her neighbor. If we are seen as gene-driven machines looking out for ourselves, the possibility of community and meaningful relationships is jeopardized by an ideology that discourages their realization. All of life is defined by competition, devoid of a genuine capacity to reach out in honest concern for the neighbor. Our society is already burdened by an excessive individualism that compromises every attempt at community building; a genocentric view of human beings accentuates that burden.

Assuming a society (looking now well into the future) in which a genetic ideology prevails and genetic enhancements have become widespread among the more affluent class, the implications for ethics would be sobering. The ethics of a society are governed by the people's vision of a good society, and that vision must capture in significant measure the interdependence of people. The sense that we need each other must be cultivated in order to establish a cohesiveness that is the mark of a healthy society. To accomplish this situation in the twenty-first century is difficult enough—at least for a secularized nation in the Western world—but one can see how the challenge would be intensified in a society where the lure of success and achievement centers on genetic enhancements. Rather than self-improvement being a goal toward which one strives, one pays the fee for a genetic "fix." It would be the worst kind of elitism, where the goals and advantages of life do not go to those who strive and attain, but to those who receive the genetic equipment that enables them to attain. A society can live with an elitism that comes from success and achievement on the part of those who have the natural endowment to excel, but can society live with an elitism based on the ability to *purchase* that natural endowment? Should society be expected to live with that kind of injustice?

What I am arguing here is the ethical importance of equality of opportunity, which is an issue of social justice. We recognize that abilities and talents differ markedly between people, resulting in wide disparities in income, wealth, and social status. But equality of opportunity requires that our life prospects depend on factors that are within our own control—what we bring to the table in terms of character, intelligence, will, motivation, and skills we have developed. Enhancement supporters argue their case by implicitly justifying the aspirations that parents have for their children. Wanting the very best for their children is seen as a desirable trait of parents, one that appears to transcend any challenge or critique. That is a mistaken assumption, however, since parents do not always act responsibly in their desires for their children. Quite easily parents become obsessed with their child's achievements, often as a way of realizing their own aspirations. For how many could enhancement be seen as no more than the self-indulgence of the affluent, engaging in a project that generates pride and status for the family? Beyond these dynamics is a still more fundamental notion introduced by Christian faith, that children are a gift from God. This implies that parental authority has limits; it does not allow for the kind of autonomy that seeks to "design" one's children. That desire turns the child into a product that belongs to the parents, rather than a gift that calls for responsible stewardship:

> Surely there are moral limits that must be placed on parental choice if its exercise is not to be in danger of commodifying children. In the prospect of genetically engineering progeny, one faces that danger in an extreme form. The human genome, in a sense the carrier of life between the generations, is an entity of such value that its manipulation is a matter of extreme ethical sensitivity. . . . Here is a case where the hackneyed phrase "playing God" may really be relevant as a moral warning.[30]

While I have pictured the drive for enhancements as a basically selfish matter, an attempt to get the edge in a competitive world, one can also see it from another perspective: the drive for perfection. One might say that what gives moral substance to the argument of enhancement advocates is that they are building their case on an admirable base: the deeply human desire to improve oneself, to become better in the pursuit of perfection. The problem, however, is the means by which one seeks to attain this goal. Whatever the context, if perfection in human life is worthy and rewarding, it is because of the struggle that has gone into it. Much of the noble and inspiring nature of the human story is to be found in the striving and effort that go into this eternal quest for excellence. For the prize to be bestowed as a result of a genetic operation upon one's body is quite the opposite, neither inspiring admiration nor providing the satisfaction of earning one's reward. Whether achieved through psychopharmacology or GE, perfection is drained of its rewarding sense of accomplishment. Enhancement advocates would challenge this argument, saying that genetic enhancement would create a superior nature with which one identifies; it is as much "me" as what I would have been without improvement. That argument assumes that nothing has changed, that memory has been wiped out, and neither the enhanced person nor society is capable of evaluating what has taken place—a frightening prospect.

Michael Sandel of Harvard University, who served on the President's Council on Bioethics, proposes a more fundamental idea in challenging the genetic quest for perfection: "We would do better to cultivate a more expansive appreciation of life as a gift that commands our reverence and restricts our use."[31] Recognizing one's life as a gift from God is an essential mark of the Christian's self-consciousness, a point I have alluded to in previous pages. But Sandel, a political scientist, argues that everyone can recognize the "givenness" of human existence, whether as a gift of God or of nature. Our advent into life and who we are is not a matter of our own choosing; we are subject to structures of life that invite and inspire an attitude of humility and a sense of solidarity with fellow human beings. This is not a fatalistic outlook that passively accepts the status quo, but an expression of realism concerning human limits that recognizes the difference between the struggle to improve ourselves and the attempt, through GE, to enhance our performance and design our children. This kind of technology, says Sandel, can be seen as "the ultimate expression of our resolve to see ourselves astride the world, the masters of our nature." It betrays a mind-set and vision that threaten "to banish our appreciation of life as a gift, and to leave us with nothing to affirm or behold outside of our own will."[32]

The President's Council on Bioethics has probed these ideas in its report *Beyond Therapy: Biotechnology and the Pursuit of Happiness.*

While one can fault the degree of alarm that runs through the report, it does convey many helpful insights. It sees the dream of perfection as paramount in the gifts promised by biomedical technology, but those gifts also relate to other desires and goals inherent to human experience and aspiration: "desires for longer life, finer looks, stronger bodies, sharper minds, better performance, and happier souls"—in short, all that we believe will improve our lot.[33] Unlike the rosy optimism seen in advocates of enhancement, the report is severely critical of this prospect, delivering some penetrating observations that reveal the questionable nature—and the hollowness—of these aspirations:

> In wanting to improve our bodies and our minds using new tools to enhance their performance, we risk making our bodies and minds little different from our tools, in the process also compromising the distinctly human character of our agency and activity. . . .
>
> In seeking brighter outlooks, reliable contentment, and dependable feelings of self-esteem in ways that bypass their usual natural sources, we risk flattening our souls, lowering our aspirations, and weakening our loves and attachments.[34]

## *Theological Concerns*

The basic issue raised by the preceding concerns is the major theme of this book: How are we to understand human nature? For people of faith, it is ultimately a theological question, because it cannot be answered without reference to our Creator. By emphasizing our relationship to God and to each other as central to whom we become as human beings, we are saying that a genocentric view of humanity fails to get at the defining character of our nature. It is our spiritual life that reveals that defining character, giving rise to the central questions of human existence: "Who are we?" and "Why are we here?" It is expressed as well in the moral life that leads us to responsible relationships with each other, the intellectual life that discovers truth through insight and discernment, and the aesthetic life that opens one to appreciation of the beautiful and the lovely. These rich realities of human experience, found within community and in our relationships with each other, point us to the meaning of human existence.

At the same time, we have recognized that human beings cannot be understood exclusively in spiritual—or moral or intellectual or aesthetic—categories. We are embodied creatures living in the natural world, and who we are is not fully understood without the knowledge that the sciences provide. When we recognize that our biological character is the foundation for our spiritual life, making it possible, we see the necessity of integrating body and spirit in a holistic unity that neither regards the body as a biological machine nor divorces the spiritual life from its biological roots. Maintaining this unity is both an affirmation of faith that sees human beings as creatures that bear the image of God and an expression of a persuasive anthropology that captures the fullness of human life and experience. As such, it enables one to respond effectively to the enhancement challenge. Scientists who espouse genetic enhancements betray a truncated view of human nature, reducing its level of explanation and understanding to the realm of molecular biology. In doing this, they fail to recognize that human nature involves a self-understanding marked by goals, intentions, and purposes that must be addressed on their own ground rather than being "explained"—and thus explained away—on the basis of physicochemical activity at the molecular level. Only with this truncated view of human nature could one imagine a program of genetic enhancement that would seek to produce a new and improved human being.

My belief is that the basis for an effective response to genetic enhancements is a different view of human nature, one that I am proposing from a Christian point of view. There are writers approaching this subject from a secular perspective who also insist that the critical issue revolves around human nature. Francis Fukuyama, for example, observes:

> Even if genetic engineering on a species level remains twenty-five, fifty, or one hundred years away, it is by far the most consequential of all future developments in biotechnology. The reason for this is that human nature is fundamental to our notions of justice, morality, and the good life, and all of these will undergo change if this technology becomes widespread.[35]

This observation raises the critical question: What kinds of changes resulting from genetic enhancements would actually constitute a threat to our human nature? Fukuyama regards notions of "justice, morality, and the good life" as inviolable, expressing what it means to be human; genetic changes could threaten those concepts as a consequence of losing our humanity. In light of the understanding of human nature presented in part one, what particular concerns do we bring to this issue of genetic enhancements?

## Human Nature and the Human Future

My answer to the preceding question lifts up our humanity as creatures in relationship with God and with our fellow human beings. I suggested that our relation to God introduces the notion of bearing God's image; we are creatures who must believe in order to find meaning and direction in our lives, whether that faith is in the Creator or in some finite and necessarily inadequate substitute in the world. If God is the ultimate reality of and for our lives, then everything else stands in relation to that fact. We would be less than human if we lost the sense of mystery inspired by our creaturely nature that directs us to God the Creator. We would be less than human if we lost the sense of living in a moral world, experiencing the moral demand and moral striving, our sense of obligation and compassion that relates us to our neighbor in responsible ways and creates human community. The experience of vulnerability, the struggle for self-improvement, the sense of guilt and of moral failure, the need of recognition and achievement, the yearning for forgiveness and reconciliation—if any or all of these features were removed from human experience, our humanity would be severely diminished or disappear.

The prospect of genetic enhancement is sufficiently theoretical that one can hardly predict whether it will ever constitute an actual threat to this description of human nature. Much of the enhancement discussion relates to increases in performance levels that are not intended to transform as much as to reach some degree of improvement in human capacities. For that reason, many advocates would argue that rather than threatening our humanity, enhancements would actually make us more human in the sense of realizing our human potential. However, it is precisely this desire to fashion a more perfect creature that prompts theological and ethical objections. The belief that we can improve the human being through GE introduces the presumption that we can engineer a more perfect being of our own making, one who would ultimately become completely "other" in the words of biologist Gregory Stock. An appropriate term to describe the quest to realize this dream is what the Greeks called *hubris*, an arrogant pride or presumption. It is not genetic manipulation in itself that warrants this charge, for it can serve a healing purpose; it is the intention to use that manipulation to produce an ideal creature.

Thus, my objection to the genetic enhancement argument is not that those marks of humanity I find to be essential will necessarily be removed, a prospect that would beggar the imagination and clearly warrant massive objection. It is, rather, the need to challenge the hubris involved in embarking on a quest that signals the disdain of God's creation, intending to create an alternative being with the ability to transcend all the faults, limitations, and weaknesses that burden human existence. Perhaps the proper response to such a quest is to ignore it because of its illusory character, but we have seen that a number of scientists seriously promulgate the idea and are intent on achieving it. Biologists including James Watson, Lee Silver, Gregory Stock, Gregory Pence, and many others should not be ignored. They are ardent enough in their advocacy to gain a fair amount of public attention, thus warranting a serious theological response.

In defining human nature, I made it a point to recognize our biological origins as a species emerging during the course of biological evolution. This evolving character of the human led me to affirm an "open-endedness" that is inherent to our nature. If this is in fact the case, should we not be open to potential changes that could result in a more enhanced species? In responding to that question, one must distinguish between biological and cultural evolution. Biologically, we do live with change, and we do not know what course biological evolution has in store for us, other than the fact that whatever changes take place will occur over a very long period of time. While our species is unique in the animal world, it is also thoroughly embedded in that world and subject to the ongoing process of evolution. Our uniqueness does not require people of faith to believe that our human nature is fixed and immutable, nor does it require them to believe that humanity is the end goal of biological evolution. It is hardly becoming of creatures to declare the end to a process that has created them, nor can we limit God to the present state of affairs. We thrive as individuals with an uncertain future, and we can also thrive as a species with an uncertain future.

In contrast to biological evolution, cultural evolution is a human creation in which we are producing significant and relatively swift changes with sophisticated tools of technology. Emerging technologies—whether the industrial machines that threaten the ecology that supports us, nuclear weapons that threaten annihilation on a massive scale, or the tools of microbiology that might change human capacities and our relationships with each other—have always posed momentous choices for the human community. In living our lives "into the future," we carry out our God-given destiny, but how we order our lives and relationships as we go forward is not simply a matter of human freedom and autonomy. Cultural evolution places a huge obligation on human societies to function responsibly and with wisdom in the way they handle the life-changing technologies at their disposal. Genetic enhancement is a technological and cultural phenomenon based on a false, reductionist view of humanity. Consequently, when enhancement advocates seek to improve the human prospect, they mistakenly believe that tampering with people's genes has to be the ultimate solution. This belief and goal ought to be repudiated on both moral and theological grounds.

Along with humanity's openness to the future, another concept relevant to this discussion is "created co-creator," a term proposed by theologian Philip Hefner. This term accentuates the creative potential of our species and could be interpreted as justifying the goals of enhancement advocates. My understanding of the concept, however, does not embrace the notion of "self-creation," which could appropriately describe the goals of genetic enhancement. This understanding would also take exception to the view that our technology will fashion a transformed human being as cyborg or *technosapien*, a creature in which the organic and technological are internally merged to make a new form or expression of the image of God. Technology is a human creation that gives new shape and direction to human life but should not be expected to redefine the human or transform humanity into a creature that no longer bears the nature and identity of *Homo sapiens*. I tend to believe that any reference to cyborgs or androids is little more than a testament to the rich imaginative powers of human beings (we are seeing the concept brilliantly exploited in novels and films), but to identify this form of "techno-nature" with the image of God is to step over a crucial line that must be maintained between God's creation and our creations. The latter can at best *serve* God's purpose rather than *becoming* God's purpose; to claim the latter invites an idolatry of its own.[36]

The adjective *created* in "created co-creator" thus signals a restriction in our capacity to bring into being what is new; it recognizes the limitations inherent to our finitude and resists any attempt to remove them. The drive to create within the human context is the drive to gain greater control over ourselves and our environment, a control that offers greater freedom to achieve the things we perceive to be desirable. That is a worthy goal in itself, but only when those pursuing it recognize that our desire for control always exceeds our capacity to achieve it. Humankind has been well served by the wisdom that can distinguish between illusory and realistic goals. Tampering with the given character of the genome in order to create a new, enhanced being is an attempt to avoid the struggle for human improvement by changing the ground rules that govern that struggle. That goal is neither realistic nor appropriate. There is also the intractable ethical factor that holds us accountable for the kind of control and mastery we seek. Even if it were possible to enhance the human genome for the generations yet to come, do we have the wisdom and insight to make that kind of decision? Could we avoid the unintended consequences that would be sure to arise?

## Concluding Thoughts

In spelling out theological objections to genetic enhancement, I have not objected on grounds of principle to every kind of genetic manipulation. I believe there is a place for the utilization of recombinant DNA in fighting genetic disease in the lives of individuals and, should it ever become a safe and viable procedure, for intervening in the germ line to effectively cure diseases that would occur in succeeding generations. I see this biomedical therapy as dictated by a compassionate concern for the sick and disabled. On the objection that one cannot distinguish between therapeutic and enhancement GE because they are integral to each other, I recognize the problem but also believe that sufficient distinction can be made to carve out a policy that would provide support for counteracting devastating genetic diseases. Without doubt, there will be attempts to practice enhancement medicine, and passing laws that make it illegal may not be realistic in every case. The task of the medical profession, which serves as a gatekeeper in a matter of this kind, is to encourage the appropriate professional organizations to adopt codes of behavior that discourage expending financial resources, time, and energy in pursuing human enhancement through GE. A serious effort would also be needed to educate the public on the implications this kind of pursuit would have for society. Issues of justice and fairness are having an impact on the subject of enhancement in the world of sports, and they are likely to have an impact in the larger society as well.

My reservations concerning genetic enhancements, assuming that the technical obstacles are eventually overcome, lie in the realm of ideas. Those who are advocating genetic enhancements display an ideology, which means here that they are promoting an agenda through the promulgation of ideas about the human future. Their ideology reveals an anthropology that I have labeled genocentric and characterized as inadequate, and it contains goals I have described as hubristic and illusory, seeking comprehensive control over the human body and its environment. In making these charges, I do not deny that those who advocate genetic enhancements are typically acting in good faith, proposing a vision of the human future in which they deeply believe. Indeed, many may see them as heroic in their confidence in the human capacity to overcome limitations and rise to a "new humanity" that brings renewed promise to the future. One must look below the surface of this drive for control and judge whether it in fact serves the human cause, whether it embodies wisdom or presumption.

One must acknowledge that some Christians argue on theological grounds that genetic enhancements are a justifiable goal. Ted Peters, for example, approaches this subject on the basis of a future-oriented anthropology, emphasizing the human as co-creator with God in fashioning "a better future." This leads him to a cautious acceptance of the possibility of genetic enhancements: "We should at minimum keep the door open to improving the human genetic lot and, in an extremely modest way, influencing our evolutionary future." This is not "playing God" but "playing human," as God intends for us.[37] Where I have focused on those scientists who are advocating dramatic enhancements and a transformed human future, reflecting a truncated, genocentric view of the human being, Peters is encouraging a cautious but more open attitude to the prospect of "beneficent" enhancements. What constitutes "beneficent" enhancements is an obvious issue here, but I believe our major concern should be to draw protective lines around the human genome. The appropriate middle ground between the opposite poles of total rejection of GE and the advocacy of genetic enhancements is the limiting of gene modification to healing catastrophic diseases. This approach would be viable when protected by ethical and legal restrictions.

Enhancement advocates often extol personal freedom, making it the basis of their appeal for the right of parents or individuals to pursue enhancement for their children or themselves. A matter of such personal interest, they claim, should not suffer the intrusion of government or any outside force. This affirmation of personal autonomy and freedom is perhaps the most powerful idea in our culture, but it needs to be challenged in this case. When a practice as consequential as genetic enhancement is on the table, it concerns all of society; our primary concern must be upholding the welfare of the community rather than ensuring advantages for what would certainly be a select few. Another factor here is that human procreation brings a marvelous genetic variation to society that we take for granted, serving as a basis for the pluralism that we experience in human relationships. The "genetic lottery" is often accused of being unfair, but it is actually profoundly egalitarian because everyone must play in it. If a substantial number of people were to tamper with the genes of their offspring, introducing choice in the appearance of each generation, the variation would diminish, and the consequences would be divisive. The wealthy would reap the "rewards" of enhancement, leaving behind a genetic underclass.

The vision of a transformed future for humanity that one finds in many boosters of genetic enhancement suggests for Christians the notion of a biological or genetic "salvation." One is led to believe that GE will rid the human body of its weaknesses and enhance the mind to levels of achievement we can scarcely comprehend. If salvation is to be found in this life, one could hardly ask for more. One is told that GE may even engineer a deeper religious commitment, and one wonders if not also a more sensitive conscience and a nobler soul! One is impressed with how a distorted view of the human being leads to a warped understanding of human potential and a misreading of the complex nature of the human being. Rather than bringing salvation, the advocates of genetic enhancement present a modern-day version of the Tower of Babel (Gen. 11:1-9), whose builders also believed their technology would enable them to reach the heights of heaven itself.

CHAPTER 6

# HUMAN NATURE AND THE QUEST FOR IMMORTALITY

One of the most remarkable developments during the past hundred years of human history has been the increasing life span. During the twentieth century in the United States, the average number of years that people lived grew from forty-nine years to seventy-eight, an increase of more than 50 percent. According to the Census Bureau, the number of Americans age one hundred or older has doubled every ten years and now stands at some eighty thousand; by 2050, the number of centenarians is expected to reach well over eight hundred thousand.[1] Many of the reasons for this "longevity revolution" are fairly obvious: better sanitation, clean water, the discovery of vaccines and antibiotics, better nutrition and greater emphasis on bodily care and fitness, and improved medical care that continues to make progress in combating such maladies as cancer and heart disease. Researchers are beginning to focus on centenarians as their numbers increase, and one of their discoveries is that people maintain a surprising degree of relative health and independence into their early nineties.

We live in a time of heightened interest in maintaining good health and adding years to our lives. The longest a human being has been known to live is 122 years, the age reached by Jeanne Calment, a Frenchwoman who died in 1997. As the trend toward longer life continues, it intensifies the question as to the upper limit of the human life span. And as the baby boomer generation enters the ranks of the elderly, increasing their numbers, there is also greater pressure on the medical and scientific establishments to address the problems inherent in aging. A prominent player in this development is the pharmaceutical industry, which anticipates a bonanza in the use of drugs designed to enhance the aging process and prolong life. The number of "anti-aging" companies that have started up since the late 1990s has been phenomenal. With products as varied as vitamin E and shark cartilage, these companies promise the seeker a life that is both longer and healthier. Among scientists engaged in the pursuit of enabling people to live longer, healthier lives, the focus has shifted from gerontology, the study of aging, to "biogerontology," indicating the impact of genetics and an expanded interest in changing what we've assumed to be the inexorable course of getting old. (A more recent coinage along the same lines is "geroscience," denoting an exclusive interest in anti-aging efforts.) Scientific centers and institutes that focus on life extension are springing up around the country, and the recently formed American Academy of Anti-aging Medicine boasts a membership of some twelve thousand physicians.

## Living with the Prospect of Death

This driving interest in human mortality, with dreams of overcoming it, has a long history going back to ancient times. A distinctive feature of human consciousness is the realization that at some point we will inevitably die. Not only are we mortal, but we *know* that we are mortal, and this fact constitutes an indelible mark on our consciousness. We live with many limitations as human beings, but none approaches the inexorability and ultimate character of our mortality. From the beginning of human history, this recognition that life means ultimately death has inspired myths of many kinds, often portraying human resistance to the prospect of our demise. From the rich store of Greek mythology addressing this topic, a particularly poignant myth is that of Tithonus, son of the king of Troy, who was loved by Aurora, the goddess of dawn.

At the request of Tithonus, Aurora secured for him the gift of eternal life, but it turned into the disaster of interminable old age. He should have requested eternal youth, not just unending years; the myth suggests that the quality of our existence, not just its quantity or length, is the real issue. The increased frailty of Tithonus finally moved Aurora to turn him into a grasshopper, a rather far cry from what he was seeking.

In addition to the mythology, history is replete with legends and stories about miraculous cures of disease and reversal of mortality itself. Medieval alchemists worked with the "philosopher's stone" that reputedly was able to turn base metals into gold, which when melted could be consumed as an elixir that would bring renewed life and immortality. From ancient times, springs have been regarded as miraculous sources of healing and renewal, as in the New Testament account of the pool of Bethsaida (John 5:2). In American history, we are familiar with the story of Juan Ponce de León, the Spanish explorer and governor of Puerto Rico, who in 1513 was supposed to have searched the present state of Florida for springwater that was thought to be a "fountain of youth." In more recent centuries, a mixture of scientific findings and the desire for a longer life has resulted in some quite bizarre solutions to the disabilities of aging. A particularly interesting one was offered in 1889 by the respected French scientist Charles Brown-Sequard, who claimed he could rejuvenate old men with a tonic containing the crushed testicles of dogs. Scientific efforts today are becoming far more sophisticated, with some promising to translate what has been a human dream into scientific reality. The subject of myth and legend is now being addressed in the laboratory.

What are possible outcomes of the aging research now in progress? One recent survey identifies four projections that are part of the current discussion:

1. *Prolonged senescence.* We will gradually increase the human life span to 150 years but spend the last 50 in frailty, depending on caretakers. This view represents the failure of life-extending efforts, and no one is advocating it. It is often presented by skeptics as the likely outcome of efforts to improve on what is now seen as the "natural" life span, and

it also serves as a foil for those who are projecting a far more promising outcome.
2. *Compressed morbidity.* This view poses an ideal in which we lead long lives free of chronic diseases and disabilities and then die quickly as we "wear out" from the aging process. The goal would be to prevent "premature" aging and the ailments associated with it. Life expectancy would increase but not significantly, within a fixed maximum life span.
3. *Decelerated aging.* There is a clear difference in viewpoint among biogerontologists on whether slowing the pace of aging is plausible and desirable; some say it is both, while others say it is neither. Those in the former camp would see future ninety-year-olds as healthy and active as today's fifty-year-olds, with a correspondingly longer life span.
4. *Arrested aging.* At the most radical end of the scale are biogerontologists who believe we can successfully reverse the damage caused by the metabolic processes that cause aging. This would result in an indefinite postponement of aging, with death likely coming from acute collapses rather than from chronic deterioration. Typical projections among those in this group would be a two-hundred- to five-hundred-year life span, and even more.[2]

As humans live longer, it is clear that, for a fortunate minority at least, relatively good health is stretching into the eighties and nineties. While the possibility is disputed among biogerontologists, it will not be surprising if better health over a longer period of time will stretch our life span to a maximum of 130 years or longer. The question posed by our interest in human nature is whether the third and fourth of the four projected outcomes have implications that should concern not only the Christian but society as a whole. What will be the psychological and sociological consequences if the life span of humans actually moves into the range of, say, two hundred or three hundred years? Are we to welcome the prospect of living "indefinitely"? Is our mortality a boundary that challenges our best efforts to overcome? We have seen how genetic engineering poses the possibility of overcoming our genetic limitations in the quest for enhanced bodies and minds; in this chapter, we examine what would have to be the most significant enhancement of all.

## The Controversial Embryonic Stem Cell

Human embryonic stem cells (ES cells) are an important part of regenerative medicine, prompting much excitement over the prospect of their use in healing genetic diseases and other disorders. But ES cells play a critical role in anti-aging efforts as well. Amid all the excitement and expectation they have created, ES cells are also a highly controversial topic because of the ethical issues raised by their use. Given the range of their importance and potential, as well as the ethical and theological issues they raise, it will be helpful first to give a brief description of stem cells and a consideration of the ethical questions raised by their use before turning to their significance for extending the human life span.

In the previous chapter, I referred to somatic cells that carry out specialized functions in the body, whether in organs or in other tissue such as muscle or bones. These adult cells are differentiated according to the particular tasks they carry out in various parts of the body, but ES cells, in contrast, are not yet differentiated; they do not carry out specialized tasks but are in a preliminary state that can lead eventually to any particular function that the body needs. As undifferentiated cells, they can replicate or self-renew themselves indefinitely through cell division, and as they differentiate to carry out specific tasks, they act as a repair system that replenishes cells that have been disabled through old age, injury, or disease. This capacity to renew or repair somatic cells is called "potency," which is further categorized as follows: *Totipotent* stem cells are identified with the zygote or fertilized egg; they can without exception grow into any type of cell. *Pluripotent* stem cells are embryonic cells that can grow into most of the two hundred or more cell types that make up the human body. *Multipotent* stem cells produce only cells of a closely related family of cells (such as the variety of cells that constitutes blood). *Unipotent* stem cells, such as the germ cells in the testes and ovaries, carry out a single function.

There are adult stem cells (AS cells) as well as ES cells, but while the latter are pluripotent, the former are typically multipotent and thus not as effective. Also, AS cells are not easily accessible from the tissue where they are found, and as they mature, their ability to change becomes increasingly limited. Unlike ES cells, they can only be grown in culture with considerable difficulty. They are currently being used in treatments for many diseases and conditions (particularly in combating blood diseases), but AS cells lack the plasticity of ES cells to form specialized cell types different from the tissue in which they reside. However, researchers continue to pursue a number of possibilities in the use of AS cells in order to avoid the ethical issue raised by ES cell research. That issue is the destruction of human embryonic life. ES cells are obtained from the undifferentiated mass of an early-stage embryo (called a blastocyst), which requires the disassembling of the embryo and its consequent destruction. If AS cells can be reprogrammed in a way that enables them to function more effectively as therapeutic agents, the destruction of ES cells could possibly be avoided. Recent research in Japan and the United States has claimed success in reprogramming human skin cells back to an embryo-like state, with no need for eggs or for embryos. It would appear that before long, the main ethical reservations concerning stem cell research may well be resolved.

Other efforts are also being made to find new ways of generating ES cells without destroying the embryo. One possible approach comes from a routine practice in fertility clinics that has been used to check the embryo's health. For years it has been known that early embryos do not seem affected by the removal of one of their virtually identical eight cells, called blastomeres. Working with mouse embryos, researchers have found that withdrawing a single blastomere and cultivating it in a dish with stem cells results in its becoming "stemmy." Apparently the chemicals involved in this procedure flick the right genetic switches in the blastomere to turn it into a stem cell. In August 2006, a biotech company in Boston, Advanced Cell Technology, announced its success in deriving stem cells through this procedure, but many scientists are dubious about the long-term promise of these efforts.

ES cell research in which the embryo is destroyed raises a critical moral question: What is the nature of human life at the embryonic stage? Answering this question brings us back to the discussion of human nature in part one. I maintained in chapter 1 that central to our understanding of human nature is our God-given capacity to relate to God as a covenantal partner and to other humans as fellow creatures. We do not become who we are as human beings without being in relationship, which is essential to the self-knowledge and self-awareness that characterize our humanity. This relational view of human nature means that we *become* human by virtue of our birth and entry into the life of relationship. Historically, this discussion has centered on abortion, where the embryo has been implanted in the womb and begins its development from embryo to fetus to birth. In this context, embryonic life is *potential* humanity, undergoing biological development that is essential to our becoming human beings. This understanding has two implications: to abort an embryo is not an act of killing or murdering a human being, but it is also more than a simple removal of tissue. This stance leads to the conclusion that abortion is always a misfortune and never to be taken lightly, but under certain circumstances it can be justified.

The situation with ES cell research poses a different ethical issue. We are again addressing embryonic life, but now it is not in the womb, destined for birth, but in the laboratory. Because of this change in context, the embryo's destruction does not raise the moral issue of abortion. Christians will disagree among themselves on this point, but Jewish tradition acknowledges its validity by not attributing legal or civil status to genetic materials outside the uterus, even if an embryo is involved; such materials lack potential humanity until they are implanted in a woman's womb.[3] Nonetheless, the embryo is more than human tissue and thus creates a particular obligation for those who would destroy it. Respect for the embryo in this context requires that its destruction can be justified only if it serves a humanitarian purpose, such as overcoming the tragedy of genetic disease or other traumas. An appropriate expression of this respect is also seen in the efforts being made—as noted earlier in this section—to utilize the embryo without destroying it or to sufficiently perfect the use of AS cells so as to make unnecessary the use of ES cells. Scientists tell us, however, that if this latter case is ever to occur, further research on ES cells will be required for the time being in order to gain the necessary understanding of cellular biology that will enable them to utilize AS cells.

Another facet of this issue that relates to the discussion in chapter 1 is the understanding of the soul. We have seen that, in spite of the Bible's holistic understanding of the human being, much of the church's theology continues to maintain a dualistic position in which we are divided into body and soul, or material and spiritual elements. When related to the beginning of life in reproduction, this is expressed in the creationist viewpoint of Roman Catholic theology, where God creates the individual soul as a separate act from the body's biological development. There has been an alternative view in the theological tradition—seen, for example, in the Protestant reformer Martin Luther (1483–1546)—called the *traducianist* view. It holds that the soul is generated from the parents and mirrors the same kind of development that occurs with the body. Both can be likened to seeds that develop over time, coming finally to fruition; a complete human being in terms of both body and soul is not present until the time of birth. This view is analogous to what today is called a developmental view, which sees a gradual becoming of the human being from potentiality to actuality, achieving one's full humanity with entry into the world.

These two views in the Christian tradition carry significantly different implications for the moral status of embryonic life. The creationist view attributes full humanity to life from the moment of conception, which means that destruction of the embryo, whether in the womb or in the laboratory, is equivalent to the killing of a human being in society. Because life is fully ensouled at conception, there is no difference in the moral value or weight of the embryo and the living person. This view obviously leads to a repudiation of abortion from the moment of conception, as well as stem cell research. In contrast, we can infer from the traducianist view and today's developmental view (which are more in tune with a psychosomatic understanding of human nature) that the moral weight of life increases from its humble beginning to a fully human life in relationship. This means that for life in the womb, the moral status of the fetus increases as it grows and nears the time of birth. Thus, in this view, destruction of embryonic life, while a serious matter, is far removed from the language of killing. This view would allow for stem cell research, but an important ethical restriction that is commonly adhered to in laboratories around the world would limit such research to the first fourteen days of embryonic life. This is when the "primitive streak" appears, or the beginnings of the central nervous system, at which point the process of biological individuation is complete. (Until then, we don't know whether one, two, or more individuals could emerge from the embryo.) More extensive government regulation is needed in this area as an expression of our respect for life in its early stages, both to ensure that research is done exclusively for the purpose of healing diseased people and to prevent the commercialization of the process.

Any reference to stem cell therapy has to acknowledge that it is still in its infancy. Much remains to be learned, many obstacles must be overcome, and there is a real danger that public expectations exceed what can be accomplished in the near future. At the same time, it is not unrealistic to believe that ES cell research will eventually revolutionize the treatment of a variety of diseases. One of the most promising possibilities is treatment of Parkinson's disease, where people have lost brain cells that create the chemical dopamine, resulting in tremors and loss of muscle control. ES cells have already been prompted to specialize into cells similar to these dopamine-creating cells. Type 1 diabetes is another disease where stem cells may be helpful, forming new islet cells in the production of insulin. Injected into the liver, they may eliminate the need for insulin injections that people with diabetes typically use today to manage this disease. If researchers can find a way to control the specialization of stem cells into any type of cell, many more diseases and injuries—liver disease, ALS, arthritis, spinal cord injuries, to name but a few—could find significant treatment. Nor can one overlook the tremendous impetus that stem cell research gives to scientists in gaining a better understanding of cellular life, including the division and differentiation of stem cells. This, in turn, will enhance the efforts of researchers in combating cancer, which involves the improper growth and differentiation of cells.

One aspect of ES cell research related to the potential use of stem cells as a therapeutic tool is cloning. The widespread controversy over this procedure relates to the cloning of an individual person, which would mean the birth of an individual who shares the same genetic heritage as another person already living in society. This has been done in the animal world—notably with the sheep named Dolly—but not among humans (in spite of a few well-publicized claims to the contrary). Opposition to the cloning of a human being is certainly understandable and justified for a variety of reasons. The real interest of scientists, however, is not to reproduce a cloned individual but to use the procedure of cloning for therapeutic purposes. A significant obstacle to the infusion of stem cells into a patient is that the immune system of the patient resists the entry of genetic material that is not one's own. To overcome this problem, biologists are working with somatic cell nuclear transfer (SCNT), which is the more exact term for cloning. When serving a therapeutic purpose, SCNT involves taking the nucleus of a somatic cell from the tissue of a diseased patient (most likely a skin cell among the millions shed daily) and inserting it into an unfertilized egg from which the nucleus has been removed, so that the DNA of the egg is now that of the patient. The egg is induced to divide and soon forms a blastocyst (a ball of approximately 150 cells), from which an embryonic cell line can be derived. This provides ES cells that can be inserted into the patient without danger of rejection, enabling them to carry out a therapeutic purpose. While this procedure is now largely theoretical for humans, it has been successfully performed with animals and is expected to eventually become a viable option for humans.

When one sees the ethical issue posed by embryonic research within the context of potential healing of diseased and suffering people, I believe the moral weight clearly lies on the side of healing people. There is no moral revulsion over the destruction of life at the embryonic level that begins to compare with the anguish and grief of witnessing the premature demise of people afflicted with a genetic disease. I can appreciate the argument that there are boundaries to what we can achieve in alleviating the pain and burden of human existence, but I am not convinced that we should draw that boundary in a way that removes the promise of healing in ES cell research. To insist that microscopic, nonsentient life must receive the exact same respect as living people is to make an intellectual distinction that lacks moral force; it does not compel a strong sense of obligation, particularly when matched with the healing promise of stem cell research. In terms of ethical theory, my conclusion here is based on teleological reasoning that says the end can justify the means: where the goal is therapeutic, embryonic research is justified. Or, putting the matter in broader context, our moral duty to heal the sick and afflicted should govern our assessment of ES cell research.

## Stem Cells, Telomeres, and the Life Span

What do ES cells have to do with the quest for immortality? We have noted that ES cells are self-renewing in that they can go through unending cycles of cell division without differentiating into a terminal state—in other words, without becoming a somatic cell. They are a tool of our body that is always there to regenerate tissue as needed. Through cloning, or SCNT, the patient's somatic cells are used to generate ES cells that can be differentiated into whatever kinds of cells the patient needs—pancreatic cells for diabetes, heart cells for a failing heart, liver cells for combating cirrhosis, and so on. This development will obviously have an effect on an increasing human life span, but the goal for some is still more ambitious. There are scientists who believe that if and when we are able to fully harness the regenerative powers of stem cells, we will be looking at the possibility of maintaining the human body indefinitely as a regenerating, self-renewing organism. They are intent on *reversing* the aging process. If the time comes when ES cells can be isolated and grown at will, these cells could theoretically become an endless source of young cells to replace those that are failing from old age.[4] This is not just the regeneration of particular organs but the beginning of "rejuvenation medicine," a term now being used to describe this heady prospect.

Scientists are pursuing other avenues of exploration in the antiaging quest, some of them coalescing with the use of ES cells. A notable representative of this pursuit is Michael D. West, a bioengineer who has written a book entitled *The Immortal Cell* describing his quest to understand and "defeat" death.[5] West observes that in the course of evolution, moving from single-celled to multicelled creatures, a change has taken place with the forming of somatic cells, which—unlike germ cells of sperm and egg—are programmed to self-destruct. In other words, aging is inherent to somatic cells, and research has shown that this aging is linked specifically to cell division rather than the general wear and tear that come with the passage of time. Given the fact that all body cells carry the same DNA as germ cells, West wondered whether there had been some kind of modification in the somatic cells—perhaps a genetic switch of some kind—that took effect millions of years before and has led to their aging and death. The question then is whether it may be possible to decipher this "clock" that is responsible for cellular aging and possibly change or even reverse it.

The pursuit of these questions has led West and other scientists to the telomere hypothesis, which was first proposed in 1971 and has become one of the major points of interest in the effort to understand and possibly change the aging process. What are telomeres? Like the rest of a chromosome and its genes within the cell nucleus, they are sequences of DNA made of the four nucleic acid bases (A, T, G, and C), but they have particular positions on the chromosome. Located at each end, they "cap" the ends of the chromosome (like the plastic tips at the ends of shoestrings), protecting them from fraying or fusing together, which would make the cell malfunction and die. In working with aging cells both in the laboratory and in the human body, scientists have observed that telomeres get shorter with the continual dividing of the cell until they are no longer able to carry out their protective function. Apparently, as somatic cell telomeres shorten to a critical stage, the cell recognizes them as damaged DNA and stops dividing, which means the onset of senescence and death. The goal of telomere research became figuring out how and why this process takes place.

In the course of this research, scientists found—for West the decisive discovery—that the telomeres in cells cultured from the male germ line remain constant in length. How, if at all, was this related to the fact that germ cells, unlike somatic cells, continue to divide and do not age? A critical breakthrough came in 1997 with the discovery of what came to be called the telomerase (tel-AHM-er-ace) gene, which is found in germ cells as well as in cancerous cells that are engaged in cellular division that never stops. Telomerase is an enzyme that adds bases to the ends of telomeres, and the question now became whether adding telomerase to somatic cells would prevent their telomeres from shortening also, thus keeping the cells dividing and halting their aging. West's team conducted an experiment with skin cells, some of which were without telomerase and some with the gene expressed. Within two months, the untreated cells began to slow down and stop, while the telomerased cells continued to function "as though they were still young. . . . We had halted the aging process of human cells!"[6] The question that was still not answered, however, was whether this success with body cells could be translated to the whole body, slowing down the process of aging in a way that was meaningful for human beings. West opines that cellular aging could constitute as little as 5 percent or as much as 90 percent of human aging. He adds, "But even if it were only five percent, and we could change that five percent, wouldn't we have done something wonderful?"[7]

After years of working with telomeres, West realized that not just the germ line but stem cells, if they could be utilized as totipotent, would themselves constitute *zoe*, the Greek term he uses for immortal life. With the arrival of Dolly the sheep, it was shown that with SCNT, a body cell could be transplanted into the environment of an egg cell to be "reprogrammed" so that it acts as an embryonic cell. The question then for West was whether, by taking old cells with short telomeres and returning them to egg cells by cloning, one could reset their telomere length. If so, the cell would in effect become young again in regard to its normal life span. In Dolly's case, such a reversal did not happen; her telomeres were prematurely short, making her about six years old at birth as far as her cell life was concerned (and Dolly did die prematurely). Scientists then began to focus on combining the activation of telomerase with nuclear transfer in an effort to produce cloned animals with full-length telomeres. Laboratory experiments at Advanced Cell Technology in Boston, where West at the time was chief scientific officer, resulted in normal-length telomeres through the action of the telomerase gene, which, they found, seemed to "awaken" in the embryo to make sure that the age of the cells was properly young. For West, this experiment was historic, signaling a profound turn in human history that eventually would reshape the future of humanity:

> For the first time in history, we have the potential to transfer the immortality of the germ line into the soma, along with

other powerful new insights into the biology of aging and disease that have the potential to build a new and brighter world only dreamt about in ancient Mesopotamia.[8]

## Other Aging Factors

According to a research team at the University of Utah, when one considers the three factors of telomere length, chronological age, and gender (women live longer than men), those factors account for 37 percent of the variation in the risk of dying among those in the over-sixty age group. What causes the other 63 percent? One major cause of dying is "oxidative stress," where oxidants, or oxygen-carrying substances that create energy in reaction with other chemicals, can damage the body's DNA as well as proteins and lipids (fatty substances that are important in the formation of the cell membrane). Normally, cells can repair this damage, but it can lead to such illnesses as atherosclerosis, Parkinson's disease, and Alzheimer's disease. Oxidation and its effects on longevity have generated many scientific studies; one series of experiments with worms exposed them to two substances that neutralize oxidants, resulting in an increase of an average 44 percent over their normal life span.[9] However, other similar experiments have proven to be inconclusive.

Another factor in aging is "glycation," which results from a sugar molecule (fructose or glucose) bonding to a protein or lipid molecule so that eventually they can no longer carry out their role. Our cooking and eating habits clearly play a decisive part in this process, as do the production practices of food companies. The sugar added to many products for human consumption comes in a form that is proinflammatory, causing body tissues to malfunction and initiating such diseases as diabetes and cancer as one grows older. Here again, scientific studies have found a possible antidote: substantially reducing caloric intake can have considerable impact in counteracting the effects of glycation. One recent study showed that genetic alteration, together with dietary restriction, can increase the life span of mice by around 70 percent. Other studies involving gene alteration have shown that the life span of nematodes (worms) can be extended from 31 to 199 days; translated into human terms, that would be a life span of some 700 years.[10] In view of the excitement that these kinds of experiments can generate, it is important to note that life extension efforts work much better in species with a short life span than in longer-lived species. We can engineer far more dramatic extensions in nematodes and fruit flies, for example, than we can in mice, a fact that would apply all the more to humans.

Another factor related to aging is the pools of adult stem cells that are located throughout the body, held in reserve to replace cells that wear out or are lost to injury or disease. These cells are finite in number, and during a lifetime, they are gradually depleted, leaving the body without the cellular reinforcement it needs. One proposed antidote to this problem would be to extract adult stem cells from the body and grow more of them, reinfusing them into the patient. Other factors as well are related to aging and senescence; these include chromosomal mutations that cause cancer and mitochondrial mutations that are linked to the production of free radicals (chemically unstable molecules that set off chain reactions leading to oxidative stress). Not surprisingly, the process of aging is quite complex. Yet the argument of those who would "defeat" death is that we are too easily mystified by that process. Biogerontologist Aubrey de Grey argues that it is not a matter of correcting *all* of the metabolic processes that are potentially damaging to one's health, but rather a matter of *fixing damage as it happens*. He likens the body to one's car, which he sees as a "strikingly exact" analogy to the human body at the cell, tissue, and organ level; replacing an organ in one's body will become as routine as replacing a fender on one's car. With sufficient maintenance, both car and body can be kept going "more or less indefinitely."[11]

This optimism of de Grey, a prominent figure in the anti-aging scene who teaches at the University of Cambridge, is based on his belief that the molecular and cellular changes associated with aging can now be attacked by the anti-aging therapies previously discussed. Demonstrating a knack for entrepreneurship, he has devised a research program called Strategies for Engineering Negligible Senescence (SENS), which he hopes will contribute significantly in gaining the financial support needed to mount a meaningful attack against the destructive effects of aging. Aging, says de Grey, should be regarded as a disease just as HIV is, summoning the same kind of commitment and governmental resources that will enable society to gradually turn it around. He deplores those who oppose anti-aging efforts, regarding them as caught in a "pro-aging trance," offering rational arguments on behalf of the irrational. He believes—naively, in the view of many—that once society recognizes what can be accomplished in the rejuvenation of middle-aged mice, extending their healthy lives by a considerable amount, people will catch the vision of life extension and will insist that the government raise taxes in order to achieve it. He estimates it would cost about $300 billion per year in the United States (an amount he claims will not bankrupt us because it is close to what our nation has spent on the war in Iraq) to keep everyone treated pharmacologically in suppressing the effects of aging.[12]

Biologist Gregory Stock agrees with de Grey that once society realizes that aging is not an inevitable process of decline, greater resources will become available and aging research will explode. Since aging is a universal phenomenon, "the most predictable health problem we face," he sees it as an ideal candidate for germ line engineering. Once we understand the genes associated with aging, we will be able to alter them in order "to inhibit, circumvent, or compensate for normal aging mechanisms,"[13] not just for our contemporaries but for generations to come. We must recognize aging as *the* disease: "It affects everyone, it cripples, it kills, it is brutal, and suddenly it would be seen as potentially treatable."[14] Advocates like de Grey and Stock see their anti-aging concerns as deeply moral, responding to the suffering and tragedy caused by the vulnerabilities of aging. They are convinced that decelerating the aging process will at the same time prevent the onset of diseases characteristic of old age, because pushing back the boundaries of aging and death will prolong the health associated with youth and middle age. This means that people will die from other causes like accidents rather than experience the suffering introduced by old age. As de Grey says, we can avoid "the Tithonus error."

## Biblical Insights on Human Mortality

In responding to scientific attempts to overcome human mortality, the Christian mind is informed by the biblical story. In chapter 1, I referred to the resurrection of the body as the New Testament's defining belief concerning human destiny, and now I must bring that belief into conversation with the subject of this chapter in shaping an appropriate response. The remaining pages will constitute a brief overview of perspectives on death and the afterlife found in the Old and New Testaments, a reflection on how we can understand the substance of those perspectives in contemporary theology, and a final critique of the quest for immortality, grounded in a Christian understanding of human nature.

In chapter 1, I argued the necessity of a holistic view of the human being that rejects the historic dualism of an immortal soul housed in a mortal body. This view affirms the prevailing stance of biblical scholars on this subject. It recognizes that death in the Old Testament is not seen as the departure of a living soul from a now lifeless body, but the loss of breath or "life force" (*nephesh*) that now ceases to animate the flesh. Whether conceived in terms of blood or breath, this life force is an impersonal energy that comes from God and dissipates at death.[15] Our mortality is simply a part of what it means to be a creature: "We must all die; we are like water spilled on the ground, which cannot be gathered up" (2 Sam. 14:14). Death is thus a fact of life and not to be seen as a riddle or absurdity. What makes a "good" death is to die in old age, surrounded by family, and to be well remembered; a "bad" death, by contrast, is one that is premature, is violent, or leaves the deceased with no surviving heir.[16] At death, one departs to the abode of the dead, *sheol*, an undesirable kind of shadow existence that is neither a heaven nor a hell but simply a part of a divinely ordered structure of things.

One of the distinctive features of Old Testament faith that accentuates human mortality is the exalted nature of God, whose eternalness stands in contrast with the transiency and impermanence of human beings. One of the most powerful expressions of this awareness is seen in Psalm 90:

> Before the mountains were brought forth,
> > or ever you had formed the earth and the world,
> > from everlasting to everlasting you are God.
> You turn us back to dust,
> > and say, "Turn back, you mortals."

> For a thousand years in your sight
> > are like yesterday when it is past,
> > or like a watch in the night.
> You sweep [mortals] away; they are like a dream,
> > like grass that is renewed in the morning;
> in the morning it flourishes and is renewed;
> > in the evening it fades and withers. (vv. 2-6)

This fragile, transitory nature of human life is not offered as a lament or a cry of desperation, but as recognition of the awesomeness of God. Because of sin, we are at times the object of God's wrath, but also of the steadfast love of God, whose presence is a source of hope and consolation for mortal beings.

An interesting question about human mortality in the Old Testament—particularly significant here in light of our subject—is whether the story of the fall in Genesis 2–3 signals the loss of a chance at human immortality. Scholars have speculated whether the punishment directed at Adam and Eve as a result of their succumbing to temptation does not indicate the thwarting of God's intent to create an immortal creature. This possibility is inferred from the fact that their punishment involves a "return to the ground" (3:19), words that denote mortality, as well as exclusion from the Garden of Eden so that they would not take fruit "from the tree of life, and eat, and live forever" (3:22). Presumably, a continuing access to the tree of life would have endowed Adam and Eve with immortality. A cross-cultural reference on this point is the Mesopotamian Epic of Gilgamesh, which, besides sharing with the Genesis story such features as food and a serpent, also lifts up the desire for immortality. However, the fact that "the LORD God formed man from the dust of the ground" (2:7) would indicate that from the beginning, God's design was that of a mortal creature who was made from dust and who would return to dust.[17] This understanding is more likely the case; the tree of good and evil rather than the tree of life plays the central role in the story, with the hubris of Adam and Eve focused on gaining knowledge that belongs to God alone, rather than a quest for immortality.

This understanding would preclude the idea that death is a punishment or curse under which humans have been placed as a result of their fallen state. One does not find this idea in subsequent Old Testament literature either, although a "bad" death such as dying prematurely could be the result of sin. But as the Old Testament scholar Lloyd Bailey observes, "mortality as the Creator's design for humans seems to be the basic perspective of the Old Testament literature," as well as Rabbinic literature.[18] This perspective begins to change in some of the Apocryphal books, written during the intertestamental period—roughly the two centuries before the birth of Christ. In the Wisdom of Solomon, for example, written in the second century B.C.E., we read (according to the New English Bible translation) that "God did not make death" (1:13) and "God created man for immortality . . . it was the devil's spite that brought death into the world" (2:23-24). This association of death with the devil or demonic powers receives more attention in the New Testament, particularly in the letters of the apostle Paul, where it actually takes on a central role. This warrants a more careful consideration of Paul's theology as we turn to the New Testament.

Understanding Paul's references to death is not a simple matter, because his use of the term moves well beyond denoting biological death. Paul uses the concept in a wide metaphoric sense to cover "everything within creation which deviates from the Creator's design."[19] When Paul says, "The wages of sin is death" (Rom. 6:23), he sees death as a manifestation of the power of sin and demonic forces that have infected the whole world. He relates sin and death to the heritage of Adam, a heritage that has prevailed in history until the appearance of the "new Adam," Jesus Christ, whose resurrection has overcome the power of sin and death (1 Cor. 15:20-22). On the basis of 1 Corinthians, death is clearly the enemy to Paul: "The last enemy to be destroyed is death" (15:26). However, when one moves from the context of theology and eschatology to that of pastoral care, and specifically to Paul's reflections on his own death, one sees a different picture. In his letter to the Philippians (written while in jail), he reveals a divided mind about his future; it would be better for his congregation if he continued on with his work, but "my desire is to depart and be with Christ, for that is far better" (1:23b). Here, as a man of faith, Paul regards death as a gateway to a fuller life with Christ.

Is death, then, a friend or an enemy for Paul? One might reply that it depends on which context one is addressing, but that would likely be seen as an attempt to paper over a contradiction in Paul's thinking. Yet I believe these two views do hold together if we look more carefully at what Paul is saying. The "sting" of death, says Paul, is sin (1 Cor. 15:56), which means death as a threat and enemy is due to our alienation from God. Sin threatens and can remove our capacity for trusting God because it moves us to seek control over our lives and destiny. This means, in turn, that death stalks us as an enemy because it is the ultimate verdict on our lives that we *cannot* control in the sense of avoiding it or preventing it from happening. What this means is that death is not inherently or necessarily an enemy, an absolute absurdity that can only confound and defeat us. Rather, our sinful state of alienation from God turns death into a fearful enemy; it becomes a void and an abyss, threatening the meaning that we seek to give to our lives and leaving us without hope.

In contrast, the resurrection faith, says Paul, holds out a promise that actually overcomes death, where "death is swallowed up in victory" (see 1 Cor. 15:54b). Where people are living this resurrection faith, death is seen through different eyes: not as a threatening void but as a gateway to a transformed life, where "this perishable body puts on imperishability, and this mortal body puts on immortality" (1 Cor. 15:54a). Paul himself clearly shares this resurrection faith, so the prospect of his own death does not pose a threat. This conviction is seen also in his assertion in Romans 8:38 that death is not able to separate us from the love of God in Christ Jesus. In a sinful world, death will always remain the enemy, but for the Christian, that sting has been essentially removed. Like *death, resurrection* is a wide-ranging term for Paul; it includes Jesus' own resurrection from the dead but also signals the defeat of death and the ushering in of a new age. Resurrection is a present reality for people of faith who now walk in "newness of life" (Rom. 6:4), but in much of Paul's discussion, as in 1 Corinthians 15, it is a future reality that Paul identifies with the end of time and the second coming of Christ. At this time, there will be a general resurrection of the dead and the inauguration of a new, transformed state: "For the trumpet will sound, and the dead will be raised imperishable, and we will be changed" (1 Cor.

15:52). The mystery of this new "state of being" compels the apostle to use paradoxical language, speaking of a "spiritual body" (1 Cor. 15:44) as a way of expressing the transformation that is to come.

We see here another tension in Paul's theology: in Philippians, he implies an immediate fellowship with Jesus when he speaks of his own death, but in 1 Corinthians, he discusses resurrection and life after death as an eschatological event, coming at the end of time. The same problem is posed by Jesus' words to the thief on the cross: "Today you will be with me in Paradise" (Luke 23:43). How do we handle this gap in time between each individual's death and a general resurrection at the end time? There is no consensus among scholars on what Paul means by his desire to "be with Christ"; some have suggested that Paul may have imagined a disembodied intermediate state between the individual's death and the end-time resurrection, but this would seriously compromise his resurrection teaching. Paul never really addresses the subject of an intermediate state, which means that it plays no role in his theology. He does not appear to see any contradiction or inconsistency between an immediate communion with Christ and a delayed resurrection, which may mean that in a postmortem world, the concepts of time and space are transcended—a notion that is well beyond our powers of imagination. What Paul certainly wants to say above all is that the God of Christian faith is the believer's Lord both in life and in death, a conviction that inspires a profound hope as we stand at the grave of a loved one or as we contemplate our own death.

For Christians, the figure of Jesus himself provides the most powerful insight into the meaning of death. His own death constitutes most eloquently the message of his life; it involved much suffering because it was horrendously violent and humiliating. In the moving scene of Jesus on the cross, one sees the depth of his struggle in his echoing the words from Psalm 22: "My God, my God, why have you forsaken me?" Jesus' death has often been contrasted with that of Socrates, who is the epitome of calmness and control as he chooses to take his life. For Jesus, death was a genuine struggle that called forth an act of submission, an act that became a model for his followers as he committed himself into the hands of God (Luke 23:46). His death as a common criminal accentuates for the Christian the depth of his suffering and, at the same time, the depth of the love that is expressed in that suffering and death. In light of the resurrection, Jesus' death on a cross literally defines the good news of God, the gospel of redemption, and as such, it reveals a paradoxical character: it is both threat and promise, both death and new life. This understanding of death in light of the cross redefines death for the Christian; its threat is never entirely removed, but it holds the promise of entry into a new life. Death as prelude to resurrection becomes a dominant theme in Christian worship in a broad metaphorical sense, including the sacrament of baptism, which ushers the Christian into the community of faith. Baptism is a "cross-like" act—dying to sin by immersion (which most graphically conveys the meaning of the sacrament) and rising to new life in Christ (Rom. 6:3ff.).

The Gospel of John presents a distinctive view of death in light of its eschatology. Rather than looking ahead to an end time, the distinction between the present and future is blurred, or telescoped into a view that scholars have called "realized eschatology" (John 1:4; 3:36; 5:24). The divine goal or end of life for the believer becomes a present reality; new life that an apocalyptic eschatology identifies with life beyond the grave becomes in John the experience of "eternal life" in the here and now. John is not denying that the believer will die in a biological sense, but the gift of God's spirit (*pneuma*) that makes all things new begins now in the believer's life. Thus, Jesus says in John's Gospel that the believer "will never die" (11:26) and has already "passed from death to life," (5:24), but this is understood in spiritual terms. John thus emphasizes the continuity in our spiritual life on both sides of the grave, and rarely is biological death mentioned. This has an impact as well on the portrayal of Jesus' attitude toward his own death, where it is not so much a "fearful ordeal to be endured" as it is a "deliberate, positive act" to lay down his life (10:17-18).[20]

This brief overview of biblical insights on death reveals variety in perspective, even within the New Testament itself, but at the same time sufficient unity so that we can glean a number of common conclusions. The fact that we are mortal beings, that life is a process that involves death, is clear enough in the pages of Scripture. Creation itself includes mortality. Our finite nature as creatures stands in contrast to the eternal nature of God the Creator, a juxtaposition that made the biblical person readier to accept death as a quite natural phenomenon. At the same time, it is also clear in the New Testament that our destiny transcends biological death, but not because we are in any way "supracreatures" in virtue of immortality that is built into our nature. As far as the human constitution is concerned, death is real, and death is final. A future life is wholly dependent upon a transformative act of God that is described as a "resurrection," a term that is used to understand the destiny of Jesus after his death and that serves as a model for understanding the believer's destiny as well. As creatures of God, we are endowed not only with qualities captured in such concepts as soul or "life force" (in the Hebrew, *nephesh*; in the Greek, *psyche*), but also with a relationship to God that is likewise captured in terms expressing the life of the spirit (*ruach*; *pneuma*). These terms don't make us immortal, but they do signal our God-relatedness and the fact that our destiny cannot be separated from the presence of God.

A critic of the New Testament vision of an immortal life in the hereafter might say that he or she sees little difference between that vision and that of the biogerontologists who propose an immortal life in the here and now. In both cases, is there not a desire to defeat death and ensure a continuing life for the individual? Several points need to be made in answering that question. Both views take the individual seriously, but they base his or her future on such entirely different grounds that the claimed similarity is superficial. The one is a faith rooted in the God of the biblical revelation, while the other is based on a claim of what biotechnology can do for us. The one is theocentric, while the other is anthropocentric. This means that the one is based on a faith that finds its end and goal in the glory of God, while the other finds its end and goal in the glory of human achievement. An adequate interpretation today of the Christian vision will readily acknowledge the mystery of the afterlife, claiming no special knowledge about what is to come. As the American theologian Reinhold Niebuhr noted in his journal, we had best refrain from talking about either the furniture of heaven or the temperature of hell. This will mean, too, that while the value of the individual is to be affirmed, that value finds its completion in the life of God.[21] The Christian concept of the afterlife is not a matter of glorifying humans, satisfying their desire for immortality as a way of getting their "due," but a matter of finding our ultimate goal in the life of God without being capable of imagining what that all means. All we can do, in trust and gratitude, is to own the mystery.

## A Critique of the Immortality Quest

The Christian recognition of the finality of death and our utter dependence upon God is far removed from many views found in contemporary Western societies. There is the secularized person who recognizes the finality of death but without a belief in God and who thus is often left in a state of anxiety concerning death and human destiny. The God-related character of human consciousness is enough to raise serious questions about the meaning of life, even among people for whom God is absent. That absence can become a void that gnaws at the desire for meaning in a threatening and often cruel world. Some find an answer to the loss of meaning by assuming the intellectual position of atheism and seeking to refute every attempt to gain a more comprehensive view of the cosmos. A related but more radical view would be nihilism, where one despairs over any attempt to carve some measure of meaning from the human experience. Others are more comfortable with a completely hands-off position, claiming to be agnostics and limiting their quest for meaning to the people and things that inhabit their world.

Those whom we address in this chapter represent a quite different kind of response. Rather than assuming a philosophical position in the face of human mortality, they are intent on using science and technology as a way of changing if not removing our mortality. They are the activists rather than the thinkers, finding in technology the ultimate answers to every threat or limitation to human happiness. Their language is at times overblown, as when they speak of "defeating" death, but whatever language they use, their goals are quite radical. Though they are not philosophers, one can discern a philosophical position lurking in the background of their program—a position with which we've become familiar in previous chapters. The case of Michael West is representative, I believe. As a bioengineer, he sees the issue from a molecular and cellular perspective, believing that the ultimate truth about *Homo sapiens* is to be found at this micro level. He concludes that human mortality is to be traced to an arbitrary development in somatic cells in which they lost the immortal character of germ cells. In his view, this would make us victims of chance, a situation that ought to be changed as soon as technology has the capability of doing it. Death in this view is an accident or an absurdity; aging itself, as the source of much pain and travail, ought not to be tolerated or endured.

The Christian alternative to this view is based on a very different narrative, one that expresses purpose and hope in the midst of life's limitations rather than understanding those limitations as the result of accident or caprice. A technology-based vision of the human future would wipe away every limitation deemed objectionable, with the assumption that human fulfillment will blossom when we realize that vision. The Christian alternative would regard that view as not only utopian but wrongheaded. Sickness and death are not absurd restrictions we are obligated in some way to abolish; on the contrary, they provide the setting for a purposeful, hopeful life that is forged in the midst of our vulnerabilities and our mortality. The self-understanding of the Christian as a child of God, living with a promise that bestows meaning to both life and death, makes the effort to extend the life span relatively meaningless. Devoting our energies to *how* we live our lives is the goal of wisdom, not trying to see *how many* years we can live by extending our lives indefinitely.

Another feature of the anti-death program is its individualism, a theme we also noted in the advocates of genetic enhancement, and certainly a prominent theme in American culture as a whole. The lead question in justifying life-extending efforts invariably centers on the wants of the individual: Wouldn't you or your child want to live longer if you were assured of continuing good health? That's a question difficult to ignore. But given the radical implications of a much longer human life span, how can such a question be asked in isolation from the larger social scene? What implications would it have for world population, for the demography of a society, and for issues of justice regarding whose lives would be extended? A major concern from a Christian perspective would be the long-term good of the society, what we often refer to as "the common good." If our relatedness in community is put at risk, then the individual-centered enhancement of whatever kind must be assessed in light of that risk. As life extension enthusiasts focus on genetic material relating to the beginning and end of the life span, they are too often oblivious to the larger psychological, sociological, and political implications of their work.

Those who have the wisdom that enables them to come to terms with their mortality—whether people of faith or not—are likely to recognize several truths. One is the fact that *death is the ultimate leveler*. Whatever the distinctions that can make a significant difference between us in this life, we are all the same in our mortality. Whether we are rich or poor, famous or infamous, known or unknown, morally upright or morally dissolute, all these distinctions do not alter the fact that we all come to our moment of death; we all ultimately meet the same end. To the wise, this is reason for humility. It is also for the wise an incentive for self-knowledge, raising questions of meaning and purpose as they relate to one's own life. In this sense, coming to one's moment of death can be a coming to one's moment of truth. The psalmist captures this thought as he contemplates his mortality: "So teach us to count our days that we may gain a wise heart" (Ps. 90:12).

Another truth to be learned is that, whether it comes sooner or later, *death is the ultimate coercer*. The unpredictability of death in terms of its cause or time of arrival for each individual can be deeply frustrating and, for some, horrendously tragic. Whether it comes early or late, death is always an arbitrary moment that carries a coercive force beyond our power to control. It is coercive in the fact that it confronts us with an ultimate boundary not of our own making or our own choosing. If we are fortunate, we can adjust to its coming and be ready to die, but the moment itself is beyond our control. This does not deny the fact that, for people of faith, the coercion of death does not make them victims; however tragic the circumstances of their death, there remains the sense of gratitude for the gift of life itself and the hope of new life in God.

Finally, *death is the ultimate socializer*. This may seem contradictory because death brings separation and loss, but it is also a powerful force in bringing us together. The prospect of death heightens our dependence upon each other, making us acutely aware that we need each other. Aging that leads to death makes us caregivers in ways that cannot be matched by any other circumstance—the closest to it would be the care of the very young. At both the beginning and the end of life, we are brought together in intensive ways in which the degree of dependence and vulnerability is unmatched. In contrast to the care of the young, however, caring for the aging person can often be a challenge to the humanity of families and society, for the conditions created by aging can change relationships, making them often difficult and burdensome. But wherever there is dependency, there is the opportunity to grow in love and compassion, fulfilling the God-given purpose of human life in loving one's neighbor. In several respects, death may well be seen as the enemy, but it is not an unmitigated evil. Whether it comes as an enemy or a friend (which it increasingly does in an aging society), it gives definition to our lives, evokes humility and wisdom in our confrontation with a universal, coercive boundary, and in our vulnerability, turns us to the life-and-death needs of each other. Thus, in the midst of our mortality, we find a deeper sense of our humanity.

## Concluding Thoughts

Throughout our conversation with those biotechnologists who are intent on removing boundaries we have regarded as natural and inherently defining of human life, we have noted their exclusive focus on molecular biology, or life at the microscopic, cellular level. My critique of this genocentric approach is that it practices a tunnel vision that does not begin to do justice to the issues it raises. The reason for this is that it constitutes a misreading of human nature, reducing the human being to a collection of material elements. In this chapter on efforts to extend the human life span, we have seen a dramatic example of this point. When Aubrey de Grey likens the human body to a car, arguing that both can be maintained "more or less indefinitely," he reveals not only a questionable anthropology but a dubious biology as well. De Grey conveys the idea that we are made up of "parts" that can wear out, and replacing them will keep us going indefinitely. This is to understand death as a medical problem that requires a medical solution, but the issue is actually far more complicated.

We can be thankful that the medical establishment works intensely at treating and preventing such maladies as cancer and heart disease, but whatever success it has is intimately linked to the life conditions encountered by the population as a whole. The current and projected improvements in medical care cannot in themselves reverse those conditions that actually *cause* early deaths—widespread poverty, malnutrition, overwork, air and water pollution, and many others. Conditions that weaken the resistance to infection and disease pose economic and political challenges that require enlightened government and effective social policies. This is where the real ethical demand comes into play, bringing the basic needs of society into focus and working for stronger and healthier communities. Life can and will be prolonged in a relatively healthy environment like our own, but to become obsessed with biotechnology as a means to postpone death indefinitely is a foolish dream that is encouraged by the kind of affluence and self-indulgence that characterizes our society. At this point, technology becomes an aid to self-denial, promoting the illusion of immortality.

This does not mean, however, that all aging research is beside the point. Michael Gazzaniga, director of the SAGE Center for the Study of the Mind at the University of California at Santa Barbara, expresses a valid point in maintaining that, since we are living longer, we should focus our efforts on diseases of the brain in order to help it keep up with our bodies:

> Dementia may simply be the result of our brains living beyond what they were designed for. If we can improve and extend their cognitive life span with stem cell or other pharmacological research, we should. . . . Helping us stay as healthy as we can until the moment of death is the proper goal of aging research—nothing more, nothing less.[22]

This emphasis appropriately focuses on the quality of one's life rather than on the quantity of one's years, on assistance to people suffering from dementia rather than on the deceleration of aging. It recognizes the crucial role of relationships in our humanity, enabling these people to continue to relate to others rather than lapse into dementia-forced isolation. It would respond directly to dire needs of people rather than push at boundaries that for good reasons appear to be intractable.

Finally, it is important to draw a connection between death as I understand it here in light of the biblical witness and the way that understanding fits with my acceptance of biological evolution. Biological death is actually part of the ongoing process in evolutionary biology; without death, there could hardly be birth without catastrophic overpopulation, which means biological birth and death are intimately connected and cannot be separated. This poses a problem for those theologians who understand Paul's words that "the wages of sin is death" to mean that biological death is the result of sin rather than built into the nature of things. On the contrary, as I have noted, it is the "sting" of death—the threatening abyss posed by death—that Paul attributes to sin and our consequent alienation from God. The overall witness of Scripture is that death is the natural conclusion to life, the God-given boundary of our creaturely existence. Because death is built into life, the mark of a mature faith is not to struggle against our mortality but to accept it. In dying, people of faith perform their final act: to freely surrender themselves to God, who is sovereign over both life and death. For the believer, to die is to commit oneself into the life of God.

# NOTES

## Introduction

1. Benjamin B. Warfield, "On the Antiquity and the Unity of the Human Race," *Princeton Theological Review* 9 (1911): 1-25. Cited in Francis S. Collins, *The Language of God: A Scientist Presents Evidence for Belief* (New York: Simon & Schuster [Free Press], 2006), 98. Some notable examples of nineteenth-century theologians using evolution as a framework for their theology are Lyman Abbott, *The Theology of an Evolutionist* (1897); John Bascom, *Evolution and Religion* (1897); and John Fiske, *Through Nature to God* (1899). The notion of a continuing creation that would at least allow for the idea of biological evolution is seen in two of the greatest giants in Christian theology, Augustine of Hippo (354-430) and Thomas Aquinas (1225-1274). See Martinez J. Hewlett, "Biological Evolution in Science and Theology," in *Bridging Science and Religion*, ed. Ted Peters and Gaymon Bennett (Minneapolis: Fortress Press, 2003), 74-75.
2. Christian response to Darwin's theory was largely influenced by several thinkers who assumed a high profile in spreading his views. Thomas Huxley in England ("Darwin's bulldog") and Ernst Haeckel in Germany (whose many works were read in the United States in translation) were ardent promulgators of Darwinian evolution, and particularly Haeckel combined it with a very explicit anti-Christian perspective. See Richard G. Olson, *Science and Religion, 1450-1900: From Copernicus to Darwin* (Baltimore: Johns Hopkins University Press, 2004), ch. 8.
3. The American Association for the Advancement of Science, in consultation with theologians, has produced a helpful book relating the theory of biological evolution to the concerns of the Christian community. See

Catherine Baker, *The Evolution Dialogues: Science, Christianity, and the Quest for Understanding* (Washington, D.C.: AAAS, 2006). Two books by Ted Peters and Martinez Hewlett also assist the religious believer in addressing the confusion surrounding biological evolution. See their *Evolution from Creation to New Creation* (Nashville: Abingdon, 2003) and *Can You Believe in God and Evolution? A Guide for the Perplexed* (Nashville: Abingdon, 2006).

4. John Polkinghorne, *Belief in God in an Age of Science* (New Haven: Yale University Press, 1998), 83. Fortunately, there are many theologians on whom one can rely and from whom one can learn in addressing the interconnections of science and theology. From the citations in the notes for each chapter, my indebtedness to such Christian thinkers as Ian Barbour, Philip Hefner, Hans Küng, Jürgen Moltmann, Nancey Murphy, Arthur Peacocke, Ted Peters, John Polkinghorne, and Holmes Rolston III, among others, is more than apparent.

## Chapter 1. The Emergent Human Being

1. I will often refer to both human nature and human identity, but the distinction between them should be noted. The former refers to our understanding of who we are as human beings, asserting what we believe to be true about the human subject, while the latter expresses our subjective awareness of ourselves. Obviously, assertions about personal identity should reflect our conclusions concerning human nature, making the terms interchangeable.
2. Cited in Arthur Peacocke, *Paths from Science towards God* (New York: Oneworld, 2001), 67.
3. Cited in Denis Alexander and Robert S. White, *Science, Faith, and Ethics* (Peabody, Mass.: Hendrickson, 2006), 75. Since the reference to Adam in Genesis 2–3 is always preceded by the definite article, it is quite possible that the ancient Israelite would have understood the story to refer to a typological "human" rather than an individual person. Later the article is dropped, as in Gen. 5:1, and *Adam* is apparently treated like a proper name.
4. Cited in Peacocke, *Paths from Science*, 179 n. 5.
5. Jürgen Moltmann, *God in Creation: A New Theology of Creation and the Spirit of God*, trans. Margaret Kohl (San Francisco: Harper & Row, 1985), 9. See Philip Clayton and Arthur Peacocke, eds., *In Whom We Live and Move and Have Our Being: Panentheistic Reflections on God's Presence in a Scientific World* (Grand Rapids: Eerdmans, 2004).

6. Peacocke, *Paths from Science*, 70. See Arthur Peacocke, *Theology for a Scientific Age*, enlarged ed. (Minneapolis: Fortress Press, 1993), 106ff.
7. Peacocke, *Theology for a Scientific Age*, 219ff. See John Polkinghorne, *Belief in God in an Age of Science* (New Haven: Yale University Press, 1998), 5ff., 94ff.
8. Kenneth R. Miller, *Finding Darwin's God* (New York: HarperCollins, 1999), 273.
9. Ibid., ch. 9. See Peacocke, *Theology for a Scientific Age*, 295ff.
10. Among these works, see Scott Atran, *In Gods We Trust: The Evolutionary Landscape of Religion* (New York: Oxford University Press, 2004); Justin Barrett, *Why Would Anyone Believe in God?* (New York: Rowman & Littlefield, 2004); and Paul Bloom, *Descartes' Baby* (New York: Basic Books, 2005). A helpful survey is offered by Robin Marantz Henig, "Darwin's God," *New York Times Magazine*, March 4, 2007, 37ff.
11. Jürgen Moltmann, "Christianity and the Values of Modernity and the Western World" (lecture, Fuller Theological Seminary, April 1996). Cited by Warren S. Brown in Warren S. Brown, Nancey Murphy, and H. Newton Maloney, eds., *Whatever Happened to the Soul? Scientific and Theological Portraits of Human Nature* (Minneapolis: Fortress Press, 1998), 225.
12. A prominent figure in the background of this discussion is the Jewish philosopher Martin Buber (1878–1965). Buber lifted up "the dialogical principle" in his influential work *I and Thou* (New York: Touchstone, 1970), stressing personal relationships and mutuality as essential marks of human existence. In authentic relationship, one "becomes an I through a You" (80). Among contemporary theologians, Douglas John Hall has given particular emphasis to the point that "human existence is co-existence." See his *Professing the Faith: Christian Theology in a North American Context* (Minneapolis: Augsburg Fortress, 1993), 323ff. Theologian Paul R. Sponheim offers a richly faceted treatment of relational theology in his book *Faith and the Other: A Relational Theology* (Minneapolis: Fortress Press, 1993).
13. This apt expression from Philip Hefner is one way to capture the twofold character of humanity in expressing both our creative capacities and our finite, limited being as mortal creatures. Hefner sees human creativity as an essential dimension of our being created in God's image. See his *The Human Factor: Evolution, Culture, and Religion* (Minneapolis: Augsburg Fortress, 1993), 27ff.
14. Philip J. Hefner, "The Human Being," in *Christian Dogmatics*, ed. Carl E. Braaten and Robert W. Jenson (Minneapolis: Augsburg Fortress, 1984), 1:330ff.

15. Warren S. Brown spells out some of the human capacities that come into play in lives marked by personal relatedness, including language, awareness of others in thought and feeling, memory, orientation to the future, and mental and emotional control of behavior. See Brown, Murphy, and Maloney, *Whatever Happened to the Soul?* 103. No one of these "capacities" defines the image of God or the humanity of the individual person, but together they serve in characterizing the person in relationship.
16. See Theodore W. Jennings Jr., "Theological Anthropology and the Human Genome Project," in *Adam, Eve, and the Genome: The Human Genome Project and Theology*, ed. Susan Brooks Thistlethwaite (Minneapolis: Fortress Press, 2003), 109ff.
17. Barbara J. King, *Evolving God: A Provocative View on the Origins of Religion* (New York: Doubleday, 2007), 212.
18. Ibid., 102.
19. John H. Relethford, *Reflections of Our Past: How Human History Is Revealed in Our Genes* (Cambridge, Mass.: Westview, 2003).
20. Ian Tattersall, "How We Came to Be Human," *Scientific American*, December 2001, 56–63. Tattersall, a paleoanthropologist, has given particular attention to the subject of human uniqueness. Two of his works are *The Monkey in the Mirror: Essays on the Science of What Makes Us Human* (New York: Harcourt, 2002) and *Becoming Human: Evolution and Human Uniqueness* (New York: Harcourt Brace, 1998).
21. A contemporary attempt by a Roman Catholic scholar to reconcile her church's understanding of the soul with biological evolution is seen in Anne Clifford, C.S.J., a theologian at Duquesne University. As an alternative to creationism, she espouses "generationism," which would understand the origin of the soul within the generative capacities of biological evolution. While this view removes the extreme dualism inherent to creationism, it still seems to imply the emergence of the soul as a spiritual entity. At the same time, Clifford refers to the soul as "a metaphorical naming of the compilation of those elements that make each of us a unique individual with a capacity for transcendence," a view that seems to express the point I am making here. See Anne M. Clifford, "Biological Evolution and the Human Soul: A Theological Proposal for Generationism," in *Science and Theology: The New Consonance*, ed. Ted Peters (Boulder, Colo.: Westview, 1998), 162–73.
22. A groundbreaking work in recognizing this fact was H. Wheeler Robinson's *The Christian Doctrine of Man*, which went through three editions and eight printings between 1911 and 1952. Robinson retained some dualistic thinking in his own theological anthropology but made the salient point

that the New Testament continues the holistic view of the Old Testament, in contrast to the dualism of Greek thought. See Joel B. Green, "'Bodies— That Is, Human Lives': A Re-examination of Human Nature in the Bible," in Brown, Murphy, and Maloney, *Whatever Happened to the Soul?* ch. 7; see also Moltmann, *God in Creation*, 255ff.

23. See Ted Peters, "Science and Theology: Toward Consonance," in Peters, *Science and Theology*, 11–39. A similar view is found in Ian G. Barbour, *Religion and Science: Historical and Contemporary Issues* (San Francisco: HarperCollins, 1997), ch. 4. For an espousal of complementarity, see Hans Küng, *The Beginning of All Things: Science and Religion*, trans. John Bowden (Grand Rapids: Eerdmans, 2007), 36ff.

## Chapter 2. Human Nature and Biological Reductionism

1. For a helpful investigation on the part of scientists and theologians representing a wide scope of converging currents in religion and science, see Ted Peters and Gaymon Bennett, eds., *Bridging Science and Religion* (Minneapolis: Fortress Press, 2003).
2. Edward O. Wilson, *On Human Nature* (Cambridge, Mass.: Harvard University Press, 1978), 192. Reissued by London: Penguin Books, 1995.
3. Edward O. Wilson, *Sociobiology: The New Synthesis* (Cambridge, Mass.: Harvard University Press [Belknap], 1975), 4.
4. Wilson, *On Human Nature*, 195.
5. Edward O. Wilson, *Consilience: The Unity of Knowledge* (New York: Knopf, 1998), 110.
6. Ibid., 55.
7. Ibid., 6. Wilson expresses this sentiment again in summarizing his argument (265): "The true evolutionary epic, retold as poetry, is as intrinsically ennobling as any religious epic."
8. Ibid., 128.
9. Philip E. Johnson, a Christian lawyer at the University of California, Berkeley, first presented the case for Intelligent Design in his book *Darwin on Trial* (Downers Grove, Ill.: InterVarsity, 1993). He has since outlined the program of ID in combating scientific materialism in *The Wedge of Truth: Splitting the Foundations of Naturalism* (Downers Grove, Ill.: InterVarsity, 2000). The principal scientific argument in support of ID is found in two books by a professor of biochemistry at Lehigh University, Michael J. Behe: *Darwin's Black Box: The Biochemical Challenge to Evolution* (New York: Free Press, 1996) and *The Edge of Evolution: The Search for the Limits*

of *Darwinism* (New York: Free Press, 2007). The mathematician William Dembski is also a prominent expositor of ID. An excellent critique from a Christian perspective is offered by the evolutionary biologist Francisco J. Ayala in *Darwin's Gift to Science and Religion* (Washington, D.C.: Joseph Henry Press, 2007). For a shorter, more popular account, see his *Darwin and Intelligent Design*, Facets Series (Minneapolis: Fortress Press, 2006). For another critique by an eminent geneticist and Christian, see Francis S. Collins, *The Language of God: A Scientist Presents Evidence for Belief* (New York: Free Press, 2006), 182ff.
10. John Polkinghorne, *Belief in God in an Age of Science* (New Haven: Yale University Press, 1998), 93.
11. See the review of Michael Behe's *The Edge of Evolution* by Joan Roughgarden, "A Matter of Mutation," *Christian Century*, October 30, 2007, 24–26. For a comprehensive treatment of these issues, see Roughgarden's book *Evolution and Christian Faith: Reflections of an Evolutionary Biologist* (Washington, D.C.: Island Press, 2006).
12. Polkinghorne, *Belief in God*, 95.
13. Arthur Peacocke, *Paths from Science towards God* (New York: Oneworld, 2001), 73–74.
14. Ibid., 75–76. A combination of contingency and providential purpose is affirmed in the Roman Catholic study *Communion and Stewardship* (2004), which received the approval of then Cardinal Ratzinger, now Pope Benedict XVI. The Catholic Church generally has been more receptive to evolution than many Protestant churches because it is not bound to a literal interpretation of biblical texts.
15. While this point can be made, it is worth noting that Arthur Peacocke is inclined to claim more than John Polkinghorne in arguing the logic of theism. He works with the notion of "the inference to the best explanation" as a way of affirming the reasonableness of theistic belief. However, what he believes can be inferred about the nature of God on grounds of scientific evidence alone is more than my own perspective (and, I believe, that of Polkinghorne) would allow. See Peacocke, *Paths from Science*, 26–30, 129–30. For an illuminating discussion of the relation of faith in God to scientific evidence, relating a fundamental, existential trust in God to rational or empirically based arguments for the existence of God, see Hans Küng, *The Beginning of All Things: Science and Religion* (Grand Rapids: Eerdmans, 2007), ch. 2.
16. For a helpful article written for laity on the developments in neuroscience, with particular reference to the brain and human consciousness, see Steven Pinker, "The Mystery of Consciousness," *Time*, January 19, 2007, 59–70.

17. Warren S. Brown, Nancey Murphy, and H. Newton Maloney, eds., *Whatever Happened to the Soul? Scientific and Theological Portraits of Human Nature* (Minneapolis: Fortress Press, 1998), 89. I have profited from the contributors to this book, sharing their concern to avoid metaphysical dualism while affirming the authenticity of the spiritual life.
18. Philip Kitcher, *The Lives to Come: The Genetic Revolution and Human Possibilities* (New York: Simon & Schuster, 1996), 283.
19. Theologian Keith Ward makes a pertinent observation concerning reductionist thinking: "The basic intellectual defect with theories of this sort is that they deny the most certain and obvious observable facts and try to replace them with very general, speculative, abstract theory." Keith Ward, *The Battle for the Soul* (London: Hodder & Stoughton, 1985), 64.
20. Gould deals with the themes discussed here in much of his work. He addresses Wilson's position specifically throughout *The Hedgehog, the Fox, and the Magister's Pox: Mending the Gap between Science and the Humanities* (New York: Harmony, 2003).
21. Gould espouses his principle of NOMA (Non-Overlapping Magisteria) as a means of overcoming "the supposed conflict" between science and religion. In maintaining the distinctive roles of these two realms as two quite different domains (he describes science as covering the empirical realm of fact and theory and religion the realm of meaning and value), Gould attributes authenticity and importance to each of them. This distinction I have espoused as well, but with an emphasis on the complementarity between the two realms and the importance and necessity of dialogue between them. Gould is more interested in removing the false understandings that create conflict between the two and resisting any effort to unify or create a synthesis between them. See his *Rocks of Ages: Science and Religion in the Fullness of Life* (New York: Ballantine, 1999).
22. Antonio Damasio, *The Feeling of What Happens: Body and Emotion in the Making of Consciousness* (New York: Harcourt Brace, 1999). Damasio addresses the false dualism in Western society in *Descartes' Error: Emotion, Reason, and the Human Brain* (New York: Penguin, 1994).
23. Antonio Damasio, interview by *The Harvard Brain*, http://www.biosynthesis.org/html/antonio_damasio.html, June 2007. Damasio provides an illuminating discussion of the mind/body problem from the perspective of a neuroscientist in his book *Looking for Spinoza* (New York: Harcourt [Harvest], 2003), ch. 5. He notes general agreement on the notion "that the mind is a process, not a thing" (283).
24. Barbara J. King, *Evolving God: A Provocative View on the Origins of Religion* (New York: Doubleday, 2007), 206–7.

25. Ibid., 207–8.
26. Cited in Hans Küng, *The Beginning of All Things: Science and Religion*, trans. John Bowden (Grand Rapids: Eerdmans, 2007), 190.
27. Pascal Boyer, *Religion Explained* (New York: Basic Books, 2001), 329.
28. Ibid., 330.
29. David J. Linden, *The Accidental Mind: How Brain Evolution Has Given Us Love, Memory, Dreams, and God* (Cambridge, Mass.: Harvard University Press, 2007), 225.
30. Andrew Newberg, Eugene D'Aquili, and Vince Rause, *Why God Won't Go Away: Brain Science and the Biology of Belief* (New York: Random House [Ballentine], 2001), 145. A related work is Andrew Newberg and Mark Robert Waldman, *Born to Believe: God, Science, and the Origin of Ordinary and Extraordinary Beliefs* (New York: Free Press, 2006).
31. Newberg, D'Aquili, and Rause, *Why God Won't Go Away*, 173–74.
32. Ibid., 176–77.
33. One sees this latter conclusion, for example, in Matthew Alper, *The God Part of the Brain* (Naperville, Ill.: Sourcebooks, 2006).
34. Nigel Williams, "Biologists Cut Reductionist Approach Down to Size," *Science* 227 (July 25, 1997): 476–77.
35. Holmes Rolston III, *Genes, Genesis, and God: Values and Their Origins in Natural and Human History* (New York: Cambridge University Press, 1999), 348.
36. Ian Barbour, *Nature, Human Nature, and God* (Minneapolis: Fortress Press, 2002), 5–6.
37. For a helpful overview of developments in this area, see Nancey Murphy, *Bodies and Souls, or Spirited Bodies?* (New York: Cambridge University Press, 2006), ch. 3.

## Chapter 3. Human Nature and the Gene

1. Ian Barbour, *Religion and Science: Historical and Contemporary Issues* (London: SCM, 1998), 226.
2. This point led scientist Robert Haynes to observe, "The genetic machinery of the cell provides the most striking example known of a highly reliable, dynamic system built from vulnerable and unreliable parts." Cited in Evelyn Fox Keller, *The Century of the Gene* (Cambridge, Mass.: Harvard University Press, 2000), 31.
3. Ibid., 54.
4. Ruth Hubbard and Elijah Wald, *Exploding the Gene Myth* (Boston: Beacon, 1999), 53–54.

5. Francis S. Collins, *The Language of God: A Scientist Presents Evidence for Belief* (New York: Free Press, 2006), 3.
6. Ibid., 125–26. The extent of the diversity or variation among human genomes is a frontier issue in genomics. As I write, there are just two individuals whose genomes have been fully sequenced: James Watson and J. Craig Venter, both notable figures in genomics. The results in regard to Venter's genome suggest significantly more variation between humans than previously recognized, closer to 0.5 percent than the 0.1 percent suggested by earlier estimates. There is an obvious reason for this difference: the researchers working with the Human Genome Project, in order to save time and money, created composite, or "reference," genomes containing only half of a human's DNA—the so-called haploid genome. Humans have a diploid genome with twenty-three pairs of chromosomes, one of each pair contributed by each of the parents. Researchers thought that working with the sequence information from just one parent wouldn't sacrifice much detail, but that has proven to be wrong. See Jon Cohen, "Venter's Genome Sheds New Light on Human Variation," *Science* 317 (September 7, 2007): 1311.
7. Collins, *Language of God*, 126ff.
8. Cited in Richard Lewontin, *The Triple Helix: Gene, Organism, and Environment* (Cambridge, Mass.: Harvard University Press, 2000), 11.
9. Ibid., 17.
10. Ibid., 17–18.
11. R. C. Lewontin, Steven Rose, and Leon J. Kamin, *Not in Our Genes: Biology, Ideology, and Human Nature* (New York: Random House [Pantheon], 1984), 273.
12. Ibid., 275. A recent argument that would support and further expand the point being made here is found in J. Scott Turner, *The Tinkerer's Accomplice: How Design Emerges from Life Itself* (Cambridge, Mass.: Harvard University Press, 2007). Turner maintains that Darwin's model of natural selection leaves the organism in too much of a passive role—at most a tinkerer—in adapting to the environment. He uses the term *homeostasis* to express the fact that organisms operate with a "feedback" mechanism that enables them to enter into the making of their environments. While Turner is not making the kind of arguments associated with Intelligent Design, he is saying that purpose and design are concepts that capture the character of organic life in its response to the environment, as well as enhance our understanding of evolutionary processes.
13. Lewontin, Rose, and Kamin, *Not in Our Genes*, 272ff.
14. Theologian Philip Hefner sees a symbiotic relationship between the genetic and the cultural in human development, co-evolving and co-adapting

together to make one reality, not two. We can speak of nature and nurture as two but only in a metaphorical way. We are the "nodal point" where these two streams come together and coexist as one, centered in the human central nervous system. Thus, there is no way of resolving the nature-versus-nurture debate, because it is based on a mistaken premise. See Philip Hefner, *The Human Factor: Evolution, Culture, and Religion* (Minneapolis: Augsburg Fortress, 1993), 29, 131.

15. See Richard C. Strohman, "Ancient Genes, Wise Bodies, Unhealthy People: Limits of Genetic Thinking in Biology and Medicine," *Perspectives in Biology and Medicine* 37 (1993): 122–44; and Walter Elsasser, *Reflections on the Theory of Organisms* (Quebec: Orbis, 1987).

16. Dean Hamer, *The God Gene: How Faith Is Hardwired into Our Genes* (New York: Doubleday, 2004).

17. Ibid., 137.

18. Ibid., 119ff.

19. Barbara J. King, *Evolving God: A Provocative View on the Origins of Religion* (New York: Doubleday, 2007), 191.

20. Holmes Rolston III, *Genes, Genesis, and God: Values and Their Origins in Natural and Human History* (New York: Cambridge University Press, 1999), 315ff.

21. Richard Dawkins, *The God Delusion* (New York: Houghton Mifflin, 2006). Recent years have seen a spate of books similar to that of Dawkins's, attacking theistic belief in the name of science. Two examples are Daniel Dennett, *Breaking the Spell* (New York: Viking, 2006); and Victor J. Stenger, *God: The Failed Hypothesis* (Amherst, N.Y.: Prometheus, 2007).

22. See biologist H. Allen Orr's perceptive review of Dawkins's book, "A Mission to Convert," *New York Review of Books* 54, no. 1 (January 11, 2007): 21–24. Alvin Plantinga, professor of philosophy at the University of Notre Dame, provides a theological response in his review, "The Dawkins Confusion," *Books & Culture: A Christian Review* 13, no. 2 (March–April 2007): 21–24. Among book-length responses, see Alister McGrath, *Dawkins' God: Genes, Memes, and the Meaning of Life* (London: Blackwell, 2004); and Kathleen Jones, *Challenging Richard Dawkins* (Louisville: Westminster John Knox, 2007).

23. Kenneth R. Miller, *Finding Darwin's God* (New York: HarperCollins, 1999), 268.

24. John Polkinghorne, *Belief in God in an Age of Science* (New Haven: Yale University Press, 1998), 10.

25. John Polkinghorne, *Exploring Reality: The Intertwining of Science and Religion* (New Haven: Yale University Press, 2005), 50ff. See his *Beyond Science* (New York: Cambridge University Press, 1996).
26. Stephen Jay Gould, *The Mismeasure of Man*, rev. ed. (New York: W. W. Norton, 1996), 359.
27. Theodosius Dobzhansky, *The Biological Basis of Human Freedom* (New York: Columbia University Press, 1956), 121–22. Cited in Rolston, *Genes, Genesis, and God*, 111.

## Chapter 4. Human Nature and the Impact of Biotechnology

1. For a helpful overview of official responses to genetic engineering on the part of churches in the late twentieth century, see Audrey R. Chapman, *Unprecedented Choices: Religious Ethics at the Frontiers of Genetic Science* (Minneapolis: Augsburg Fortress, 1997), ch. 2.
2. *Encyclopedia of Bioethics*, rev. ed. (New York: Simon & Schuster Macmillan, 1995), 1:283.
3. Eric S. Grace, *Biotechnology Unzipped: Promises and Realities*, 2nd ed. (Washington, D.C.: Joseph Henry Press, 2006), 140.
4. Ibid., 68.
5. Ira Flatow, *Present at the Future: Candid and Controversial Conversations on Science and Nature* (New York: HarperCollins, 2007), 153–54.
6. The material in these two paragraphs on nanotechnology is drawn primarily from ibid., ch. 16.
7. Ethical concerns are expressed in the increased attention being given to the need of governmental regulation of assisted reproductive technologies. Not only safety considerations but also the excesses driven by commercialism are a concern. The issues are discussed in a series of five essays in *Hastings Center Report* 37, no. 4 (July–August 2007), 16–31.
8. Gregory Stock, *Redesigning Humans: Our Inevitable Genetic Future* (New York: Houghton Mifflin, 2002), 55.
9. Cited in Bryan Appleyard, *Brave New Worlds: Staying Human in the Genetic Future* (New York: Penguin Putnam, 1998), 125.
10. Michael S. Gazzaniga, *The Ethical Brain: The Science of Our Moral Dilemmas* (New York: HarperCollins, 2006), 73.
11. Ibid., 78.
12. The material on DARPA is drawn from chapter 2 of Joel Garreau, *Radical Evolution: The Promise and Peril of Enhancing Our Minds, Our Bodies—and What It Means to Be Human* (New York: Random House, 2005).

13. Wyatt Andrews, "Medicine's Cutting Edge: Re-growing Organs," *CBS News*, March 23, 2008, http://www.cbsnews.com/stories/2008/03/22/sunday/main3960219.shtml.
14. Lee M. Silver, *Remaking Eden: Cloning and Beyond in a Brave New World* (New York: Avon, 1997), 8, 15.
15. Ibid., 125ff.
16. James Martin, *The Meaning of the 21st Century* (New York: Penguin Group [Riverhead], 2006), 195.
17. Ibid., 223ff.
18. Ray Kurzweil, *The Age of Spiritual Machines: When Computers Exceed Human Intelligence* (New York: Viking, 1999). Kurzweil addresses the prospect of a this-worldly human immortality in Ray Kurzweil and Terry Grossman, *Fantastic Voyage: The Science behind Radical Life Extension* (New York: Penguin [Plume], 2004).
19. Garreau, *Radical Evolution*, chs. 3–6.
20. Since the 1970s, a number of groups have formed that avidly pursue and promote the vision denoted here as the Heaven scenario. Perhaps most notable is the World Transhumanist Association, whose title would tell us that we are entering a posthuman age even now. Transhumanists see a growing impact of the GRIN technologies and enthusiastically welcome their promise in shaping a new direction in human history, marked by "designer children," enhanced cognition, metabolic makeovers, and anti-aging medicine, all of which will radically alter human nature. A visit to their Web site provides an insight into the flavor of this group.
21. A particularly eloquent voice in the debate over biotechnology has been Leon Kass, a University of Chicago professor and chair of the President's Council on Bioethics. Kass's view has much in common with Garreau's Hell scenario in the sense that he is pessimistic about the outcome of a biotech future. He recognizes the desire to conquer disease, relieve suffering, and prolong life as part of the humanistic vision that has always been united with the pursuit of knowledge. But he argues that these positive aspirations, when united with the immense power of biotechnology to alter and control all aspects of human life, will take on a power and momentum that will be impossible to control. Biotechnology, like technology as a whole, is not simply an instrument that we can order and regulate as we desire, because technology is ubiquitous, becoming "an entire way of being in the world." Kass brings many perceptive insights to this topic, but to my mind, his apprehensions concerning biotechnology are overdrawn. See his *Life, Liberty, and the Defense of Dignity: The Challenge for Bioethics* (San Francisco: Encounter, 2002).

22. Gilbert C. Meilaender, *Body, Soul, and Bioethics* (Notre Dame, Ind.: University of Notre Dame Press, 1995), 27.
23. Grace, *Biotechnology Unzipped*, 95.

## Chapter 5. Human Nature and Genetic Engineering

1. Audrey R. Chapman and Mark S. Frankel, eds., *Designing Our Descendants: The Promises and Perils of Genetic Modifications* (Baltimore: Johns Hopkins University Press, 2003), 4.
2. As I write, the media are reporting the world's first entirely handcrafted chromosome, using high-speed DNA synthesizers that produce genetic material from basic chemical building blocks: sugars, nitrogen-based compounds, and phosphates. While "synthetic biology" is a promising development for medicine, the excitement at this time centers around its use in industry, using cells as metabolic machines to produce ethanol, hydrogen, and other exotic fuels for vehicles. Rick Weiss, "Changing Life as We Know It," *Washington Post National Weekly Edition*, January 21–27, 2008, 6–7.
3. Chapman and Frankel, *Designing Our Descendants*, 7. The correction of various genetic defects in mice has been done for several decades now, but even here, with currently available techniques and tools, "the added genetic material is integrated with only a very low efficiency," and the genetic correction in the resulting zygote and subsequent generations "is incomplete, inefficient, and unstable." See Theodore Friedmann, "Approaches to Gene Transfer to the Mammalian Germ Line," in Chapman and Frankel, *Designing Our Descendants*, 43.
4. Cited in Lee M. Silver, *Remaking Eden: Cloning and Beyond in a Brave New World* (New York: Avon, 1997), 211.
5. One example among several of successful gene therapy took place in the early 1990s, when a young woman from suburban Cleveland, the victim of a failed immune system, was cured by the alteration of defective genes in her white blood cells. The progress of gene therapy received a critical blow in 1999, when Jesse Gelsinger, an eighteen-year-old with a rare metabolic disorder, died after receiving an experimental gene therapy at the University of Pennsylvania. Then, in 2007, a thirty-six-year-old woman, Jolee Mohr, afflicted with rheumatoid arthritis, died soon after participating in a research project in which her right knee was injected with genetically altered viruses. These tragedies emphasize the need for still more stringent protections, but unfortunately, first subjects will always face situations where not every risk can be totally eliminated.

6. David B. Resnick, Holly B Steinkraus, and Pamela J. Langer, *Human Germline Gene Therapy: Scientific, Moral, and Political Issues* (Austin, Texas: R. G. Landes, 1999), 100.
7. Ramez Naam, *More Than Human: Embracing the Promise of Biological Enhancement* (New York: Random House [Broadway], 2005), 52. Naam is a particularly enthusiastic booster of enhancement medicine and sees a significant opportunity "to sculpt our personalities" through GE, including alterations that would affect thrill-seeking and novelty-seeking behavior, mating behavior, homosexual orientation, and even strength of religious belief (55).
8. C. Ben Mitchell, Edmund D. Pellegrino, Jean Bethke Elshtain, John F. Kilner, and Scott B. Rae, *Biotechnology and the Human Good* (Washington, D.C.: Georgetown University Press, 2007), 142–43.
9. If enhancement medicine were to become a part of the expanded expectations of medical care in our society, it would raise serious issues concerning an affordable national health care policy. This is an urgent issue in itself, but it lies beyond the scope of my discussion here. A prominent voice in this debate has been Daniel Callahan of the Hastings Institute, who has forcefully argued on behalf of a sensible vision for health care that would help to curb the public appetite for ever-expanding medical services. See his *What Kind of Life: The Limits of Medical Progress* (New York: Simon & Schuster, 1990) and *Setting Limits: Medical Goals in an Aging Society* (New York: Simon & Schuster, 1987). For an opposing view, see Robert L. Barry and Gerard Bradley, eds., *Set No Limits: A Rebuttal to Daniel Callahan's Proposal to Limit Health Care for the Elderly* (Chicago: University of Illinois Press, 1991).
10. Gregory Stock, *Redesigning Humans: Our Inevitable Genetic Future* (Boston: Houghton Mifflin, 2002), 195.
11. Ibid., 197.
12. Ibid., 110.
13. President's Council on Bioethics, *Beyond Therapy: Biotechnology and the Pursuit of Happiness* (New York: HarperCollins, 2003), 35.
14. Stock, *Redesigning Humans*, 113.
15. Ibid., 155.
16. Ibid., 173. The molecular biologist Lee Silver, who is well known for his ideology of human improvement, is much bolder than Professor Stock in spelling out the features of genetically enhanced beings. Using his special language to denote the "enriched" class, in contrast to the rest of the population, he makes the following projection: "If the accumulation of genetic knowledge and advances in genetic enhancement technology continue at

the present rate, then by the end of the third millennium, the GenRich class and the Natural class will become . . . entirely separate species with no ability to cross-breed, and with as much romantic interest in each other as a current human would have for a chimpanzee." See Silver, *Remaking Eden*, 7.
17. Stock, *Redesigning Humans*, 188.
18. Gregory Stock and John Campbell, eds., *Engineering the Human Germline: An Exploration of the Science and Ethics of Altering the Genes We Pass On to Our Children* (New York: Oxford University Press, 2000), 143.
19. John Harris, *Clones, Genes, and Immortality* (New York: Oxford University Press, 1998), 203.
20. Gregory E. Pence, *Re-creating Medicine: Ethical Issues at the Frontiers of Medicine* (New York: Rowman & Littlefield, 2000), 97.
21. Cited by Lee Silver, "Reprogenetics: How Reproductive and Genetic Technologies Will Be Combined to Provide New Opportunities for People to Reach Their Reproductive Goals," in Stock and Campbell, *Engineering the Human Germline*, 59.
22. Pence, *Re-creating Medicine*, ix, 2.
23. Ibid., 105–6.
24. Richard C. Lewontin, "The DNA Era," *GeneWatch* 16, no. 4 (July 2003). Available on the Web site of the Council for Responsible Genetics, http://www.gene-watch.org/genewatch/articles/16-4lewontin.html.
25. Ruth Hubbard and Elijah Wald, *Exploding the Gene Myth* (Boston: Beacon, 1999), 162.
26. Resnick, Steinkraus, and Langer, *Human Germline Gene Therapy*, 14.
27. Hubbard and Wald, *Exploding the Gene Myth*, 64.
28. Resnick, Steinkraus, and Langer, *Human Germline Gene Therapy*, 90. See Dorothy Nelkin and M. Susan Lindee, *The DNA Mystique: The Gene as a Cultural Icon* (New York: Freeman, 1995).
29. Richard Dawkins, *The Selfish Gene* (New York: Oxford University Press, 1989), 2.
30. John Polkinghorne, *Exploring Reality: The Intertwining of Science and Religion* (New Haven: Yale University Press, 2005), 161–62.
31. Michael J. Sandel, *The Case against Perfection: Ethics in the Age of Genetic Engineering* (Cambridge, Mass.: Harvard University Press, 2007), 127.
32. Ibid., 99–100.
33. President's Council on Bioethics, *Beyond Therapy*, 21.
34. Ibid., 300.
35. Francis Fukuyama, *Our Posthuman Future: Consequences of the Biotechnology Revolution* (New York: Farrar, Strauss and Giroux, 2002), 82–83.

36. Philip Hefner uses the language of *cyborg* in this way, reflecting his concern to invest technology with a "depth dimension" that gives it theological meaning. He argues that otherwise, we run the real risk of becoming alienated from our technology and will all the more likely misuse it and suffer the consequences. I can appreciate his intention, but to understand the emerging "techno-nature" as God's new creation of cyborg, who bears the image of God, is to blur the distinction between human and divine creation and risk the danger of bestowing divine sanction on (at least in part) a "product" of human technology. The opaqueness of techno-nature makes it difficult to imagine the nature of a cyborg; is he half human, half machine? And what does that mean? The concept does not really invite rational investigation, because it belongs in the imaginary world of science fiction. See Philip Hefner, *Technology and Human Becoming* (Minneapolis: Augsburg Fortress, 2003), esp. ch. 6.
37. Ted Peters, *Playing God? Genetic Determinism and Human Freedom* (New York: Routledge, 1997), 144. See also Ronald Cole-Turner, *The New Genesis: Theology and the Genetic Revolution* (Louisville: Westminster John Knox, 1993).

## Chapter 6. Human Nature and the Quest for Immortality

1. Constance A. Krach and Victoria A. Velkoff, *Centenarians in the United States: 1990*, Current Population Reports Special Studies (Washington, D.C.: Census Bureau, July 1999), http://www.census.gov/prod/99pubs/p23-199.pdf.
2. Eric T. Juengst et al., "Biogerontology, 'Anti-aging Medicine,' and the Challenges of Human Enhancement," *Hastings Center Report* 33, no. 4 (2003): 21–30.
3. Elliot N. Dorff, "Stem Cell Research—a Jewish Perspective," in *The Human Embryonic Stem Cell Debate: Science, Ethics, and Public Policy*, ed. Suzanne Holland, Karen Lebacqz, and Laurie Zoloth (Cambridge, Mass.: MIT Press [Bradford], 2001), 91.
4. For an example of this viewpoint, see Stanley Shostak, *Becoming Immortal: Combining Cloning and Stem Cell Therapy* (Albany, N.Y.: SUNY Press, 2002).
5. Michael D. West, *The Immortal Cell: One Scientist's Quest to Solve the Mystery of Human Aging* (New York: Doubleday, 2003).
6. Ibid., 123.
7. Ibid., 129.

8. Ibid., 211.
9. Lee J. Siegel, "Are Telomeres the Key to Aging and Cancer?" *Learn.Genetics*, Genetic Science Learning Center, University of Utah, n.d., http://learn.genetics.utah.edu/content/begin/traits/telomeres/, accessed February 2008.
10. David Gems, "Is More Life Always Better? The New Biology of Aging and the Meaning of Life," *Hastings Center Report* 33, no. 4 (2003): 31.
11. Aubrey de Grey, *Ending Aging: The Rejuvenation Breakthroughs That Could Reverse Human Aging in Our Lifetime* (New York: St. Martin's, 2007), 45.
12. Ibid., 321.
13. Gregory Stock, *Redesigning Humans: Choosing Our Genes, Designing Our Future* (New York: Houghton Mifflin, 2002), 83.
14. Ibid., 85.
15. Lloyd R. Bailey Sr., *Biblical Perspectives on Death* (Philadelphia: Fortress Press, 1979), 45.
16. Ibid., 48ff.
17. Ibid., 36ff. See Jaime Clark-Soles, *Death and the Afterlife in the New Testament* (New York: T&T Clark, 2006), 13.
18. Bailey, *Biblical Perspectives on Death*, 38.
19. Ibid., 88.
20. Ibid., 95.
21. While I do not share the conceptualities of his process theology, there is much to appreciate in Norman Pittenger's treatment of our subject here. See his *After Death: Life in God* (London: SCM, 1980).
22. Michael S. Gazzaniga, *The Ethical Brain: The Science of Our Moral Dilemmas* (New York: HarperCollins, 2005), 22, 26.

# INDEX

abortion, 43
Adam, 9, 12, 168n3
aging: and current research, 138–40; as disease/absurdity, 152, 160–61; and telomere hypothesis, 148–50
anthropic principle, 10
atheism, 72–74
Augustine, 6, 16, 26
Ayala, Francisco, 172n9

Barbour, Ian, 51–52, 58–59, 168n4
Behe, Michael J., 171n9
Bible: and creation story, 5–7, 20; and human mortality, 152–60
biological evolution: and Christian theology, 5–13; and religion, 13–15
biological reductionism, xvii, 33–35, 51–54, 84
biotechnology: definition of, 85–88; and future scenarios, 100–103; impact of, 89–93
Boyer, Pascal, 47
Buber, Martin, 169n12

Callahan, Daniel, 180n9
Chapman, Audrey R., 177n1
Clifford, Anne, C.S.J., 170n21
cloning: reproductive, 97, 145–46; therapeutic, 145–47
Cohen, Lloyd, 118
Collins, Francis S., 63, 172n9
Crick, Francis, 57, 60
cultural evolution, 71–72, 76–77

Damasio, Antonio, 44
D'Aquili, Eugene, 48–49
Darwin, Charles, xii, 5, 40, 64, 82
Dawkins, Richard, 32, 71–75, 123–24
death: as life's boundary, 162–63; and resurrection, 156–59
Descartes, René, 26, 52
"designer drugs," 92
DNA (deoxyribonucleic acid), 9, 21, 57–60, 62–63
Dobzhansky, Theodosius, 5, 76

epigenetics, 68
evolution. *See* biological evolution

fertility industry, 91–92
Fukuyama, Francis, 128–129

Gazanniga, Michael, 94–95, 164
genes: and "genocentrism," xvii, 120–22, 163; and questions about, 59–62; and the "selfish gene," 71, 123–24
genetic engineering: and drive for perfection, 125–26; and genetic enhancement, 96, 111, 114–19; and genetic "salvation," 135; and genetic therapy, 108–9, 111–13; and the market system, 117–18; and social justice, 124–25; somatic and germinal, 108–110; and theological concerns, 127–35
genetics: history of, 55–59; and reductionism, 65–67
genomics, 62, 107
God: as Creator, 5–9; and genetics, 69–71; and intelligible belief, 10, 74, 82
Gould, Stephen Jay, 43–44, 75–76, 173n21
de Grey, Aubrey, 151–52, 163

Haeckel, Ernst, 167n2
Hall, Douglas John, 169n12
Hamer, Dean, 69–71
Harris, John, 118
Haynes, Robert, 174n2
Hefner, Philip, 131, 168n4, 169n13, 175–76n14, 181–82n36
Hood, Leroy, 63
Hubbard, Ruth, 61–62, 121
Huether, Gerald, 45
Human Genome Project, xv, 62–65, 107, 123

human nature: and biological evolution, 20–23; as biological machine, 52–53, 89; and the body-self, 45–46, 83; and body/soul dualism, 23–27, 29–30, 83–84, 144; and holism, xvii, 31, 52–54, 68, 122, 153; and the image of God, xvi, 10, 12–13, 16–18, 85, 129; and mortality, 137–41, 152–60; as "open-ended," 130–31; and the primates, 20–22; and relationships, 10, 15–20, 83, 142–43
Huxley, Thomas, 41, 167n2

"image of God." *See* human nature
Intelligent Design, 37–40, 73

Jeeves, Malcolm, 43
Johnson, Philip E., 171n9

Kass, Leon, 178n21
Keller, Evelyn Fox, 60–61
King, Barbara J., 19–20, 45, 71
Kingsley, Charles, xiii
Kitcher, Philip, 43
Küng, Hans, 168n4, 172n15
Kurzweil, Ray, 99–101

Lewontin, Richard, 66–67, 120–21
Linden, David J., 47
Luther, Martin, 16, 144

Martin, James, 98–99
Meilaender, Gilbert, 104–5
memes, 71
Mendel, Gregor, 56
Miller, Kenneth R., 74
Mivart, George Jackson, 24
Moltmann, Jürgen, 8, 15–17, 168n4

Murphy, Nancey, 168n4, 174n37

Naam, Ramez, 118, 179–80n7
nanotechnology, 89–90
nature vs. nurture debate, 67–68
neo-Darwinism, 20, 76
neurotheology, 48–50
Newberg, Andrew, 48–49
"nonreductive physicalism," 43

Origen, 6

Paley, William, 39
panentheism, 7–8
Peacocke, Arthur, 40–41, 168n4, 172n15
Pence, Gregory, 118–19, 130
Peters, Ted, 134, 168nn3–4
pharmaceutical industry, 92–93, 138
pharmacogenomics, 92
Polkinghorne, John, xvi, 40–41, 74–75, 168n4, 172n15
President's Council on Bioethics, 126–27
psychopharmacology, 113–14

regenerative medicine, 95–96, 141
religion. *See* science and religion
reproductive technology, 90–92
Resnick, David, 122
Robinson, H. Wheeler, 170–71n22

Rolston III, Holmes, 51, 168n4

Sandel, Michael, 126
science and religion: and complementarity of, 3–4, 28–29, 39–40, 173n21; and history of, xiii–xiv
scientific materialism, 32–37, 41–46, 84
Silver, Lee M., 96–97, 130, 180n16
soul: and creationism, 144; and reconceptualizing of, 23–27; and traducianism, 144
Sponheim, Paul R., 169n12
stem cell research, 141–47
Stock, Gregory, 92, 116–18, 130, 152

technology. *See* biotechnology
Temple, William, 7
Turner, J. Scott, 175n12

Venter, J. Craig, 175n6
Vinge, Vernor, 99

Ward, Keith, 173n19
Warfield, Benjamin, xiii
Watson, James, 57, 130, 175n6
West, Michael D., 147–50, 160–61
Wilson, Edward O., 32–37, 72, 75
World Transhumanist Association, 178n20

www.ingramcontent.com/pod-product-compliance
Lightning Source LLC
Chambersburg PA
CBHW071916290426
44110CB00013B/1379